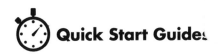

Quick Start Guides

The Essential
Low FODMAP Diet
COOKBOOK

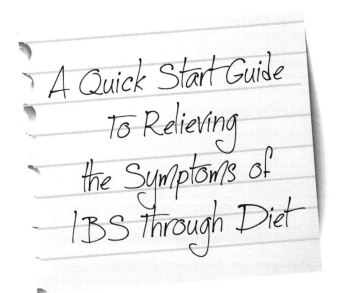

A Quick Start Guide To Relieving the Symptoms of IBS Through Diet

Improve Your Digestion, Health And Wellbeing, *PLUS* over 75 IBS Friendly Recipes!

First published in 2015 by Erin Rose Publishing

Text and illustration copyright © 2015 Erin Rose Publishing

Design: Julie Anson

ISBN: 978-0-9928232-8-3

A CIP record for this book is available from the British Library.

DISCLAIMER: This book is for informational purposes only and not intended as a substitute for the medical advice, diagnosis or treatment of a medical physician or qualified healthcare provider. The reader should consult a physician before undertaking a new health care regime and in all matters relating to his/her health, and particularly with respect to any symptoms that may require diagnosis or medical attention.

While every care has been taken in compiling the recipes for this book we cannot accept responsibility for any problems which arise as a result of preparing one of the recipes. The author and publisher disclaim responsibility for any adverse effects that may arise from the use or application of the recipes in this book. Some of the recipes in this book include nuts and eggs. If you have an egg or nut allergy it's important to avoid these. It is recommended that children, pregnant women, the elderly or anyone who has an immune system disorder avoids eating raw eggs included in any recipe.

CONTENTS

Recipes

Desserts, Sweet Treats & Snacks

INTRODUCTION

If you have been suffering from a functional gut disorder like IBS and are struggling to find the cause of your symptoms then the low FODMAP diet may be the breakthrough you have been looking for. A low FODMAP diet has helped many people to bring harmony back to their digestive system and put an end to the pain and discomfort they have endured for too long.

To help you get started, this book provides you with the essential information you need in a straightforward, easy-to-follow way which will enable you to take charge and successfully manage your condition.

In this **Quick Start Guide** you will learn which foods to avoid and which foods you can eat, discover how the diet works and how to identify your triggers, with plenty of useful tips and lots of delicious low FODMAP recipes. You'll be able to quickly implement your new way of eating with mouth-watering ideas for breakfast, lunch, dinner, desserts and treats meaning that you won't feel like you're missing out on anything.

Ready for the challenge? Let's get started.

What Is the Low FODMAP Diet?

FODMAP is an abbreviation for *Fermentable Oligosaccharides, Disaccharides, Monosaccharides And Polyols* which have been found to be common triggers found in everyday foods and can cause digestive problems. These are carbohydrates which some people find hard to digest which cause the notoriously unpleasant symptoms of IBS.

The low FODMAP diet was researched and developed by an Australian team, Dr. Sue Shepherd and Dr. Peter Gibson at Monash University in Melbourne. They found that a low FODMAP diet, a diet low in foods containing particular sugars, was capable of bringing relief of functional gastrointestinal problems in patients with IBS and other gastrointestinal symptoms. Since then the low FODMAP diet has gone global and been adopted my dieticians and doctors worldwide as a suitable way to manage gut symptoms.

High FODMAP foods are basically carbohydrates which are difficult to digest, and end up passing through the intestines to the colon because either they can't be digested, or they break down too slowly and can therefore cause discomfort and IBS. The low FODMAP diet is about reducing the amount of FODMAPs in your diet, not avoiding them entirely. Following a low FODMAP diet involves two stages, one where you eliminate certain foods and two, where you systematically reintroduce them when the time is right. A diet low in these starches may help alleviate your symptoms and bring your digestion under control to help you feel well again.

How Do FODMAPs Cause IBS?

The symptoms and severity of IBS vary from person to person, but all sufferers agree it's unpleasant. For those who struggle to digest foods which are high in FODMAPs they can have, bloating, cramps and gas because the gut bacteria respond to being fuelled by the carbohydrates passing through their intestine. As the stomach and intestines experience this difficulty, water can be drawn into the intestines. This can cause diarrhoea due to the contraction of the intestinal muscles, plus these carbohydrates provide a banquet for the natural gut bacteria to feast on which triggers fermentation and gas. The effect on the gut bacteria and the gas produced affects not just the lower part of the gastrointestinal system but can also result in a distended abdomen and bloating. The symptoms can vary in degree depending on how much of a trigger food has been consumed and your reaction to it. And that is despite many of the high FODMAP foods being healthy and nutritious whole foods. Who knew that healthy eating could be so tricky?

FODMAP foods fall into different categories and one meal is likely to contain a combination of them. The effect of consuming these starches is also cumulative, so your body may tolerate a small amount but if you increase your intake or consume it for the second time that day or in combination with another high FODMAP item, it could trigger your symptoms. For this reason it's important to follow an exclusion diet for sufficient time before carefully reintroducing a potential trigger. You can still have variety in your diet and get all the nutrients you need. Being a vegetarian on a low FODMAP diet can be particularly tricky and also if you have other restrictions to your diet, so then help from a dietician or nutritionist can really help. Remember, following a low FODMAP diet isn't forever and when you notice an improvement you can expand on the list of foods you can tolerate.

Symptom Checker

If you suffer from persistent symptoms and haven't been to the doctor for a diagnosis that should be the first thing you do. If the cause of your problems remains unknown, you may benefit from a low FODMAP diet for the following symptoms:

- Abdominal pain and discomfort
- Bloating
- Pain
- Constipation
- Diarrhoea
- Wind/gas
- Heartburn
- Sudden urgency to go to the toilet

RED FLAGS

If you have any of the following you must see your doctor immediately.

- Blood in stools
- Fever
- Unexplained weight loss
- Persistent pain
- Heartburn for more than 3 weeks

How To Get Started On A Low FODMAP Diet

If you've had recurrent digestive troubles the chances are you've already visited your doctor, but if your symptoms are fairly recent it's worth visiting your doctor, who may wish to perform tests, before you embark on a change of diet. However, if you've had IBS for some time and have tried many things to cure or alleviate the distressing symptoms, you may wish to just get started straight away.

Many people find that alcohol, caffeine and excessive fat consumption can irritate their digestion so they are best avoided or reduced as far as possible when you begin your low FODMAP diet. When you begin a low FODMAP diet the aim is to alleviate your symptoms and this will be more difficult if you're regularly consuming excessive alcohol or caffeine as these are also known IBS triggers.

There are two stages to following a low FODMAP diet. First is the exclusion phase where you avoid foods which are high in FODMAPS and the second stage is where you begin to reintroduce foods in small amounts and discover what you can and can't tolerate. The aim is to tailor your diet to your specific needs by identifying what you can and can't eat, safe in the knowledge that you can eat a wide variety of foods without problems. Some of you may already have identified some problem foods which you have already excluded so the prospect of eliminating further foods isn't exactly welcome, but please remember you don't need to stay on this forever. Plus, you can still eat healthily and enjoy your meals.

Phase 1 - Elimination

- Start by eliminating all of the high FODMAP foods listed on the following pages, bearing in mind this is temporary. The aim is to alleviate your symptoms by excluding these potential trigger foods.

- Once you remove high FODMAP foods from your diet you may notice a significant change very quickly, but for others the improvements can take longer.

- Stick to the diet for 4-8 weeks, depending on how soon your symptoms clear and you feel confident enough to try challenge foods. Often people notice an improvement fairly quickly but at the very least avoid the high FODMAP foods for 2 weeks. However, it could take as long as 8 weeks for your digestion to settle completely.

- When you are sure your symptoms are under control, move onto Phase 2.

Phase 2 - Reintroduction

If you have stuck to the low FODMAP diet for at least a month and haven't seen any improvement, you need to speak to your doctor or a dietician to discuss taking a different approach. While not everyone benefits from following a low FODMAP diet, the majority of people do see improvements.

- Once you've seen a sustained improvement in your symptoms, you can carefully reintroduce a half-size portion of one new food from one of the food groups.

- For instance you may wish to try out lactose if you've been missing dairy produce.

- Don't eat any other high FODMAP foods until you are certain that you do or do not have a reaction. Assess your symptoms over 2-3 days.

- If the test food doesn't trigger symptoms, you can try increasing the portion size, or try another food from that or another group.

- If you do get a flare up of symptoms from the test food, return to the low FODMAP foods and allow your symptoms to settle before testing another food. You can either test the same food again but in a smaller portion or continue to avoid it and try a food from a different category.

- Your tolerance can change so challenge yourself occasionally with a small amount of high FODMAP foods to add variety to your diet.

- While identifying and assessing your triggers and tolerance level, keep it simple at first then expand your range of foods, but do it systematically by only sampling one thing at a time.

- Try to leave 2-3 hours between servings of fruit to allow your body to deal with one food before introducing another. A portion of fruit is considered to be one piece and when it comes to berries, no more than a handful.

- If you have known food allergies, anaphylaxis or are coeliac, it's important to continue to abstain from the food which causes the problem. Following a low FODMAP diet involves reducing your intake of these naturally occurring sugars and it needn't be gluten-free as small amounts may do no harm. However this isn't the case if you are coeliac as it's vital to continue being completely gluten-free.

Your Food Diary

Many of us quickly eat a meal on the go and barely register what it is we've just eaten. Sometimes it's hard to remember what you had for dinner last night which makes it difficult to know what triggered off your symptoms. Keeping a food diary will not only help you keep a record of everything you eat, but it will show you what foods are causing digestive issues. You may find that you can eat a small portion of a high FODMAP item but if eaten within an hour of something else it could collectively be too much for you.

What To Record In Your Food Diary

For the duration of the elimination phase of your diet, keep a record of your symptoms. Monitor things like bowel habits, pain and bloating. Here is an example of what you can record. You can also rank the reaction on a scale of 1-10, based on severity of symptoms after eating (1 being fine, 10 being severe). Using the following examples keep a daily diary which will help you to assess how you are responding to the low FODMAP diet.

Elimination Stage		
Week	**Symptom**	**Score 1-10**
Monday		
Tuesday		
Wednesday		
Thursday		
Friday		
Saturday		
Sunday		

Once your symptoms are under control and you are beginning the reintroduction phase, keep a record of what food you reintroduce and note the quantity. Then log what, if any, symptoms you experience. Based on your reaction and tolerance to the challenge foods you should know what has caused the return of your symptoms. For example if you experience a flare up of pain, excessive wind or change to your bowel habits you'll be able to identify which food has caused it.

Reintroduction Phase		
Food & Quantity	**Symptoms**	**Reaction 1-10**
Day		
Breakfast		
Lunch		
Dinner		
Snacks		
Drinks		

The FODMAP groups containing HIGH FODMAPS are:

Oligosaccharides		Di-saccharides	Mono-saccharides	Polyols
Fructans	Galactans	Lactose	Fructose	Sugar alcohols
Wheat Barley Rye Spelt Garlic Onions	Legumes: Beans Chickpeas Lentils	Cow's milk, sheep's milk and goat's milk and dairy produce with a high lactose content e.g. soft cheeses	Apples Cherries Mangoes Pears Watermelon Honey Agave syrup High fructose corn syrup	Stone fruits such as peaches, nectarines and plums. Apples Pears Cauliflower Mushrooms Sweeteners: Maltitol Xylitol Soribitol Mannitol

Remember to only reintroduce a single food item at a time and select a food from one particular group. You could find that it is foods in one particular category which you have a problem with. If you are confident that you can tolerate a food in one category you can then expand into other foods in that category.

High FODMAP Foods List

The following foods are HIGH in FODMAPs so AVOID these.

High FODMAP Fruits

- Apples
- Apricots
- Blackberries
- Boysenberries
- Cherries
- Figs
- Lychees
- Mangoes
- Nectarines
- Peaches
- Pears
- Persimmon
- Plums
- Prunes
- Watermelon

High FODMAP Vegetables

- Artichokes
- Asparagus
- Cauliflower

- Cabbage
- Chicory
- Dandelion greens
- Garlic and garlic powder
- Scallions/spring onions (white part only, green part is fine)
- Leeks
- Mange tout (snow peas)
- Mushrooms
- Okra
- Onions and onion powder
- Peas
- Shallots
- Sugar snap peas

High FODMAP Legumes

- Baked beans
- Chickpeas (garbanzo beans)
- Black-eyed peas
- Adzuki
- Fava
- Kidney beans
- Lentils
- Mung beans
- Pinto beans
- Soya beans
- Split peas

High FODMAP Dairy Produce

- Milk, full-fat, skimmed or semi-skimmed
- Buttermilk
- Condensed milk
- Evaporated milk
- Ice cream
- Milk powder
- Milk chocolate
- Yogurt
- Cream cheese, cottage cheese, crème fraiche, mascarpone, ricotta, processed cheese and cheese spread

High FODMAP Sweeteners & Sugars

- Agave syrup/nectar
- Corn syrup
- Fructose
- High fructose corn syrup
- Honey
- Sugar free products like chewing gum, mints and sweets which contain;
- Isomalt
- Maltitol
- Mannitol
- Sorbitol
- Xylitol

High FODMAP Grains & Cereals

- Barley
- Bulgur wheat
- Couscous
- Rye
- Wheat
- This also means avoid products which are wheat based, like pasta, noodles, cakes, biscuits and breakfast cereals

High FODMAP Nuts

- Cashew nuts
- Pistachio nuts

Drinks

- No more than 1 glass of beer or wine. Alcohol is an irritant and can trigger IBS
- Dandelion tea
- Chicory coffee substitute
- Sugary drinks containing fructose or high fructose corn syrup and artificially sweetened drinks, except those using stevia, aspartame, saccharine.

Condiments & Other

- Avoid products containing inulin, fructooligosaccharides (FOS) and oligofructose. These are often found in supplements, snack bars and readymade food.
- Readymade products containing onion or garlic powder such as gravy, stock cubes (broth), salad dressings and sauces. Beware of processed meats, sausages, burgers and veggie burgers as they may contain powdered onion and garlic.

Low FODMAP Food Alternatives

The following foods are LOW in FODMAPs so they can be eaten freely.

Low FODMAP Fruit

- Bananas
- Blueberries
- Cantaloupe melon
- Cranberries
- Grapefruit
- Grapes
- Honeydew melon
- Kiwi Fruit
- Lemons
- Limes
- Mandarin oranges
- Passionfruit
- Papaya
- Pineapple
- Raspberries
- Rhubarb
- Strawberries
- Tangerines
- Tomatoes

Portion sizes of fruit:

1 piece of whole fruit e.g. banana

1 slice pineapple or honeydew melon

1 small handful raspberries

Approximately 20g (¾ oz) of a low FODMAP dried fruit

Low FODMAP Vegetables

- Alfalfa sprouts
- Aubergine (Eggplant)
- Avocados
- Bamboo shoots
- Bean sprouts
- Carrots
- Courgette (zucchini)
- Chilli peppers
- Chives
- Cucumber
- Ginger
- Green beans
- Lettuce
- Olives
- Pak Choi (Bok Choy)
- Parsnips
- Peppers (bell peppers)
- Potatoes

- Pumpkin
- Spinach
- Spring onions/scallions (green part only)
- Squash (except butternut squash)
- Sweet potato/yams
- Turnip
- Watercress

Low FODMAP Nuts & Seeds (maximum 1 handful)

- Almonds
- Flaxseeds
- Chia seeds
- Brazil nuts
- Hazelnuts
- Macadamia nuts
- Pecan nuts
- Pine nuts
- Pumpkin seeds
- Sesame seeds
- Sunflower seeds
- Walnuts

Low FODMAP Dairy & Non-Dairy Alternatives

- Almond milk
- Butter
- Coconut milk
- Coconut yogurt
- Lactose free milk & milk products
- Rice milk
- Soya milk (not from whole-beans but fine if from extract)
- Sorbet
- Whipping cream (heavy cream)

Low FODMAP Cheeses

- Brie
- Camembert
- Cheddar
- Edam
- Emmental
- Feta
- Gorgonzola
- Gouda
- Mozzarella
- Parmesan
- Pecorino
- Provolone cheese
- Romano cheese
- Stilton
- Swiss cheese

Low FODMAP Grains

- Amaranth
- Arrowroot
- Cornmeal
- Cornflour
- Buckwheat
- Coconut flour
- Gluten-free cereals, pasta and bread
- Millet
- Oats
- Polenta
- Potato flour
- Quinoa
- Rice
- Rice flour
- Rice noodles
- Sago
- Sorghum
- Tapioca
- Teff flour
- Xanthum gum

Low FODMAP Sugar & Sweetener

- Brown sugar
- Caster sugar
- Glucose
- Icing sugar
- Maple syrup
- Molasses
- Rice syrup
- Saccharine
- Stevia
- Sucrose (cane sugar, table sugar) in moderation

In Moderation Only

The following foods can usually be tolerated in the quantities shown.

- Avocado (¼ only)
- Beetroot (½ only)
- Broccoli (up to 100g)
- Brussels sprouts (up to 50g)
- Butternut squash (up to 50g)
- Celery (less than 5cm piece)
- Cottage cheese (up to 50g)
- Crème fraiche (up to 50g)
- Cream cheese (up to 50g)
- Fennel (up to 100g)
- Fruit juice of a low FODMAP fruit up to 120ml (4fl oz) per serving
- Pomegranate (½ fruit only)
- Ricotta cheese (up to 50g)
- Sweetcorn (max ½ cob)

Aside from the alternatives listed in the food you can eat, you can also include protein from fish, poultry, meat and eggs into your diet.

When you're reading product labels, gluten-free usually means wheat-free however a product may not contain gluten or wheat, but it could contain other high FODMAP foods. Always read the labels bearing in mind the ingredients are listed in descending order with the highest quantity coming first.

Tips For Low FODMAP Eating

Dealing with IBS symptoms and embarking on a change of diet can be daunting, especially if you've already been trying to eliminate various potential triggers. Aside from being aggravated by certain foods, stress can be a factor in IBS so try to make things easier for yourself. Here are a few tips to help you begin. You may be keen to find relief from your symptoms and wish to get started straight away.

- Stock up on a few store cupboard essentials and familiarise yourself with the FODMAP foods list.

- Check out what is in your cupboards and have a look at the ingredients lists on sauces, stock, gravy, chutneys and dressings Often onions or onion powder has been added.

- If you are eating out look for restaurants which can cater for specific dietary needs. A restaurant which caters for gluten-free could offer you more choice, with a menu containing less wheat products.

- Be vigilant about reading labels. Accidentally breaking your diet could cause a flare up of your IBS.

- Reintroduce foods when you feel you are ready. This could be after 2 weeks if you feel your digestive symptoms have improved sufficiently or 8 weeks if your digestive symptoms have been severe.

FAQ's

Why am I allowed some dairy products and not others?

It's to do with the lactose content. Some dairy products contain less lactose than others and milk and soft cheeses contain more than hard cheeses like parmesan and cheddar. Generally the higher the fat content of a diary product the lower the lactose content, which is good news for those who don't want to abstain from dairy products completely.

I've read conflicting information about what foods are high in FODMAP's. Why is this?

Research into the FODMAP content of foods is ongoing and for up to date information see the Monash University Website for the latest information on the FODMAP diet. ***http://www.med.monash.edu/cecs/gastro/fodmap/diet-updates/***

I am diabetic. Is the low FODMAP diet suitable for me?

It is wise to seek advice from a professional. Any changes to your diet should be undergone with the approval of your doctor and the help from a registered dietician who is familiar with the low FODMAP diet. Many doctors and clinics support it and they should be able to provide you with a list of registered dieticians, or search for one in your area.

Can I Eat Out?

Yes, although you'll need to take extra care with this especially during the elimination stage. Breaking your diet could cause an unwelcome flare up and set you back. Look for restaurants that cater for special dietary requirements. Phone ahead and explain your needs.

Recipes

Low FODMAP Cooking

A low FODMAP diet can provide for your nutritional needs and where possible we've included alternatives to the FODMAP foods you need to avoid. There are plenty of good quality non-dairy alternatives to milk which can be added to recipes, cereals or as a suitable creamer for drinks. These also have a long shelf life so once you've found one which you like you can stock up.

Without onions and garlic in your diet you may be thinking mealtimes could lack flavour and your favourite meals may be off limits, at least temporarily. However we've included recipes which are packed with tasty and healthy eating suggestions. Chives are a great way to add oniony flavour to dishes. Asafoetida is used in Indian cookery and has a distinctive pungent aroma similar to onions and garlic, so if you are really missing that flavour you could try adding a little asafoetida to curries. When using readymade stock, check that it doesn't contain onion powder or other high FODMAP ingredients. We've provided recipes for homemade stock if you can't find a suitable alternative in the shops.

Hard cheeses have a lower lactose content than soft cheeses and are suitable for a low FODMAP diet. For pizza and pasta meals you can find gluten-free substitutes which don't include wheat, just check that they don't contain other high FODMAP ingredients. Small amounts of wheat can usually be tolerated but avoid completely if you are coeliac.

By cooking your own meals with whole foods you'll know exactly what has gone into your dishes. Some people find that although they can't tolerate garlic they are fine with a little garlic-infused oil. These can be shop bought or try flavouring your cooking oil with a clove of garlic by heating the oil at the beginning of cooking, adding a whole, peeled clove of garlic and removing it from the oil after a minute or so.

BREAKFAST

Courgette (Zucchini) & Carrot Frittata

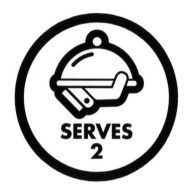

SERVES
2

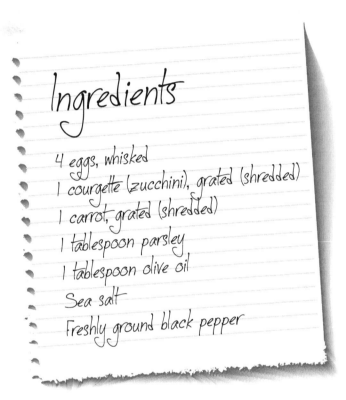

Ingredients

4 eggs, whisked
1 courgette (zucchini), grated (shredded)
1 carrot, grated (shredded)
1 tablespoon parsley
1 tablespoon olive oil
Sea salt
Freshly ground black pepper

Method

Heat the olive oil in a frying pan, add the carrot and courgette (zucchini) and cook for
3 minutes until softened. Pour in the beaten eggs. Sprinkle in the parsley and season with
salt and pepper. Allow the eggs to set then transfer to a hot grill (broiler) and cook until
slightly golden.

Blueberry Porridge

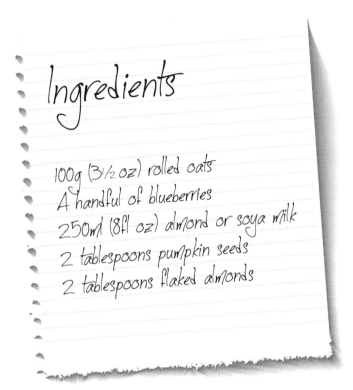

Ingredients

100g (3½ oz) rolled oats
A handful of blueberries
250ml (8fl oz) almond or soya milk
2 tablespoons pumpkin seeds
2 tablespoons flaked almonds

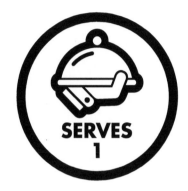

SERVES 1

Method

Place the oats and milk in a saucepan. Bring to the boil and cook for 5 minutes until it thickens. Serve topped off with the blueberries, pumpkin seeds and almonds.

Herby Scrambled Egg

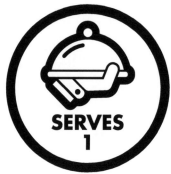

SERVES 1

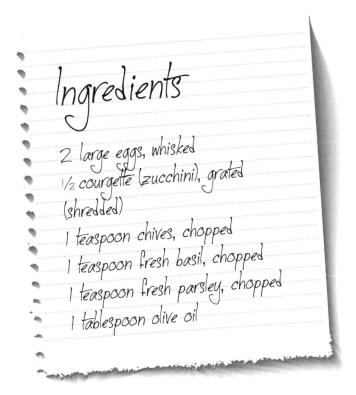

Ingredients

2 large eggs, whisked

½ courgette (zucchini), grated (shredded)

1 teaspoon chives, chopped

1 teaspoon fresh basil, chopped

1 teaspoon fresh parsley, chopped

1 tablespoon olive oil

Method

Heat the oil in a frying pan, add the courgette (zucchini) to the pan and cook for 2 minutes. Combine the chopped herbs with the beaten eggs, pour into the pan with the courgette and stir the mixture until it's lightly scrambled. Season and serve.

Chicken & Tomato Omelette

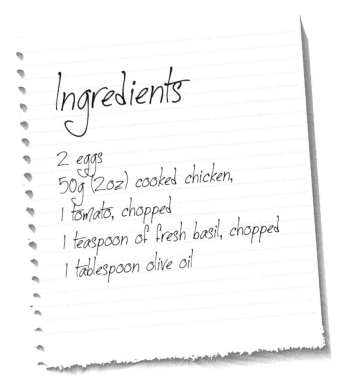

Ingredients

2 eggs
50g (2oz) cooked chicken,
1 tomato, chopped
1 teaspoon of fresh basil, chopped
1 tablespoon olive oil

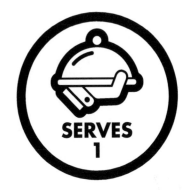

SERVES 1

Method

Put the eggs in a small bowl and whisk. Stir in the basil, chicken and tomato. Warm the oil in a small frying pan and add the beaten egg mixture. Cook for 1 minute and allow it to start to set without stirring. Continue cooking until the eggs are set firm.

Mini Meatloaves

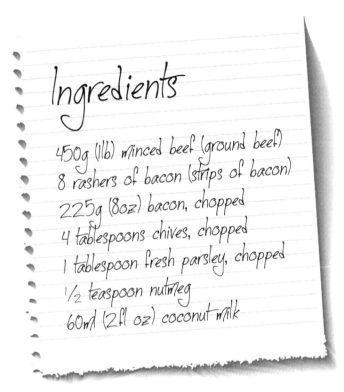

Ingredients

450g (1lb) minced beef (ground beef)
8 rashers of bacon (strips of bacon)
225g (8oz) bacon, chopped
4 tablespoons chives, chopped
1 tablespoon fresh parsley, chopped
1/2 teaspoon nutmeg
60ml (2fl oz) coconut milk

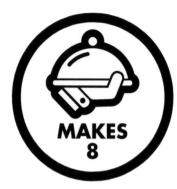

MAKES
8

Method

In a large bowl, combine the minced beef, chopped bacon, nutmeg, parsley, chives and coconut milk. Mix well. Use an 8-hole muffin tin and line each hole with a strip of bacon. Spoon the beef mixture on top of the bacon. Transfer them to the oven and bake at 200C/400F for 30 minutes. Remove the mini meatloaves from the muffin tin and serve.

Granola

Ingredients

225g (8oz) oats
60g (2 ½ oz) pecan nuts, chopped
60g (2 ½ oz) desiccated (shredded) coconut
60g (2 ½ oz) brazil nuts, chopped
60g (2 ½ oz) almond flakes
60g (2 ½ oz) sunflower seeds
60g (2 ½ oz) dried banana chips, chopped
2 tablespoons maple syrup
2 tablespoons coconut oil or olive oil
3 tablespoons water
1 teaspoon cinnamon
½ teaspoon ginger

Method

Place the oats, coconut, sunflower seed and nuts into a bowl and mix well. In a separate bowl combine the oil, maple syrup, cinnamon, ginger and water. Add it to the dry ingredients and combine. Scatter the mixture onto a baking tray and bake in the oven at 190C/375F for 30 minutes, until crisp and golden. Remove and allow it to cool. Add the banana chips. Store in a container, ready to use. Serve with non-dairy milk, such as almond, soya, oat or rice milk and a handful of fresh berries.

Wheat-Free Pancakes

SERVES 2

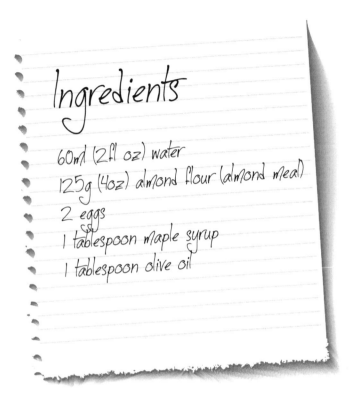

Ingredients

60ml (2fl oz) water
125g (4oz) almond flour (almond meal)
2 eggs
1 tablespoon maple syrup
1 tablespoon olive oil

Method

Whisk all the ingredients together in a bowl and make a smooth batter. Heat the oil in a pan and pour in some of the batter mixture to whatever size pancakes you require. Cook for around 3 minutes until bubbles appear and the underside is golden then turn them over to complete cooking. Repeat for the remaining pancake mixture. Serve with additional maple syrup or your favourite topping.

Coconut & Banana Pancakes

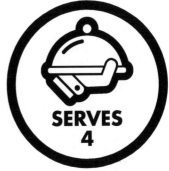

SERVES 4

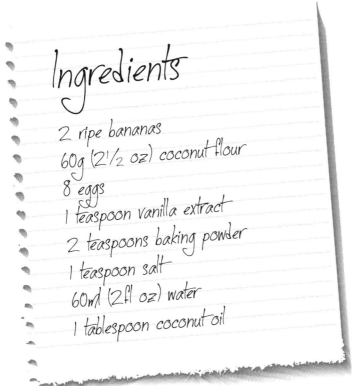

Ingredients

2 ripe bananas
60g (2½ oz) coconut flour
8 eggs
1 teaspoon vanilla extract
2 teaspoons baking powder
1 teaspoon salt
60ml (2fl oz) water
1 tablespoon coconut oil

Method

In a bowl, combine the banana, eggs, water and vanilla. In a separate bowl combine the baking powder, coconut flour and salt. Add the egg mixture until smooth. Heat a tablespoon of oil in a pan and add a little of the pancake mixture. Cook for a few minutes until slightly golden underneath. Turn it over and cook until golden. Repeat for the remaining pancake mixture. Serve with maple syrup, bacon or berries.

Blueberry & Coconut Smoothie

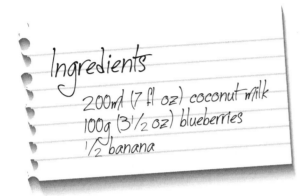

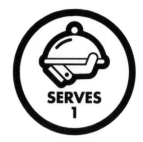

SERVES 1

Method

Toss all the ingredients into a blender and blitz. Pour and enjoy!

Carrot & Orange Smoothie

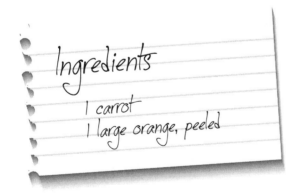

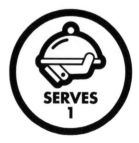

SERVES 1

Method

Place the carrots and orange into a blender and add enough water to cover them. Process until smooth.

Strawberry & Lime Smoothie

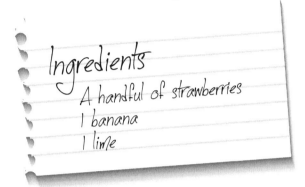

Ingredients
- A handful of strawberries
- 1 banana
- 1 lime

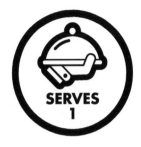

SERVES
1

Method

Place the strawberries and banana into a blender with enough water to cover then blitz until smooth. Squeeze in the lime juice and stir. Enjoy.

Raspberry & Carrot Smoothie

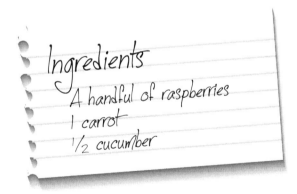

Ingredients
- A handful of raspberries
- 1 carrot
- 1/2 cucumber

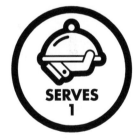

SERVES
1

Method

Place the ingredients into a blender with enough water to cover it and process until smooth.

Tomato & Carrot Smoothie

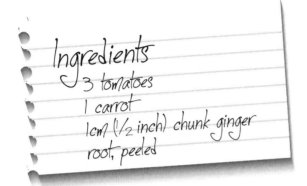

Ingredients
- 3 tomatoes
- 1 carrot
- 1cm (½ inch) chunk ginger root, peeled

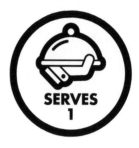

SERVES
1

Method

Place the ingredients into a blender with sufficient water to cover them. Blitz until smooth.

Strawberry & Spinach Smoothie

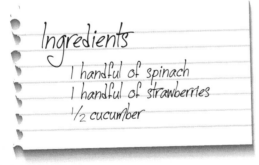

Ingredients
- 1 handful of spinach
- 1 handful of strawberries
- ½ cucumber

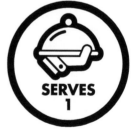

SERVES
1

Method

Place the ingredients into a blender with enough water to cover and process until smooth.

Baked Eggs & Smoked Salmon

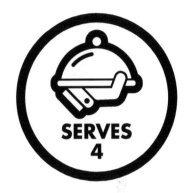

SERVES 4

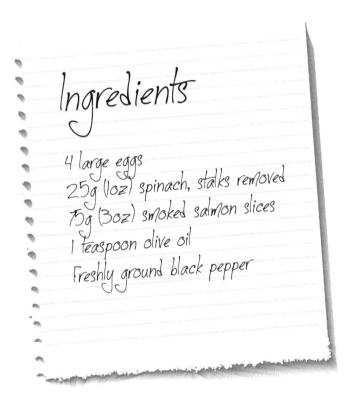

Ingredients

4 large eggs
25g (1oz) spinach, stalks removed
75g (3oz) smoked salmon slices
1 teaspoon olive oil
Freshly ground black pepper

Method

Heat the olive oil in a pan and add the spinach. Cook for 2 minutes until the spinach has wilted. Line the bases and sides of 4 ramekin dishes with smoked salmon. Divide the spinach between the ramekin dishes then break an egg into each one. Sprinkle with black pepper. Place the ramekins in a preheated oven at 220C/425F for 15 minutes, until the eggs are set. Serve and enjoy.

Hash Browns

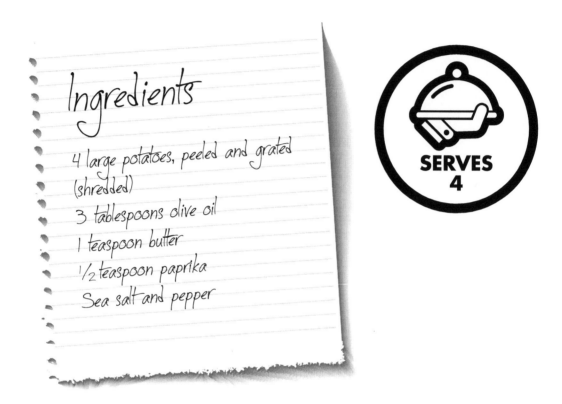

Ingredients

4 large potatoes, peeled and grated (shredded)
3 tablespoons olive oil
1 teaspoon butter
1/2 teaspoon paprika
Sea salt and pepper

SERVES 4

Method

Heat the oil and butter in a frying pan and add the potatoes. Stir and cook until the potatoes are cooked and golden brown. Alternatively shape them into patties before adding them to the pan. Add some extra butter and/or oil if you need to. Season with paprika, salt and pepper and serve.

LUNCH

Carrot & Sweet Potato Soup

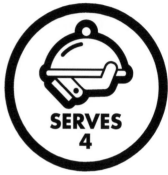

SERVES 4

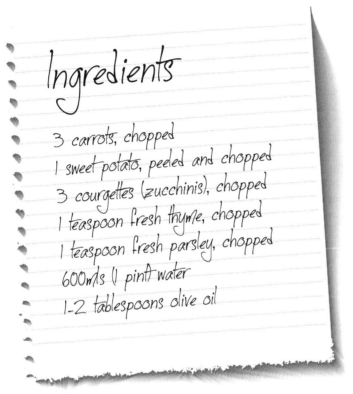

Ingredients

3 carrots, chopped
1 sweet potato, peeled and chopped
3 courgettes (zucchinis), chopped
1 teaspoon fresh thyme, chopped
1 teaspoon fresh parsley, chopped
600mls (1 pint) water
1-2 tablespoons olive oil

Method

Heat the olive oil in a saucepan, add the vegetables and cook for 5 minutes. Add the water and cook for around 25 minutes, or until the vegetables are soft. Stir in the herbs. Use a hand blender or food processor and blitz until smooth. Season and serve.

Piri Piri Chicken

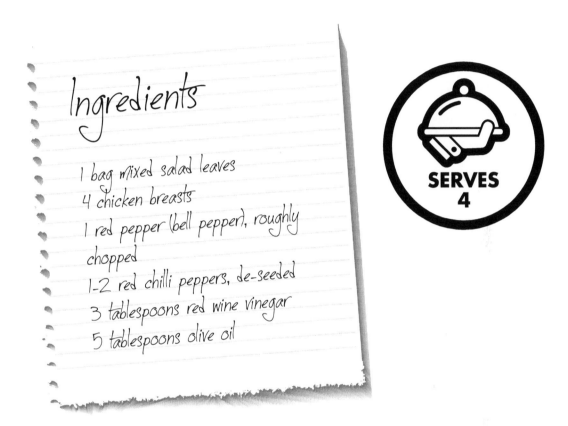

Ingredients

1 bag mixed salad leaves
4 chicken breasts
1 red pepper (bell pepper), roughly chopped
1-2 red chilli peppers, de-seeded
3 tablespoons red wine vinegar
5 tablespoons olive oil

SERVES
4

Method

Place the red pepper (bell pepper) and chillies into a blender with the vinegar and 4 tablespoons of olive oil. Process lightly leaving the mixture roughly chopped. Spoon the mixture onto the chicken and marinate for 20 minutes or longer if you can. Heat a tablespoon of olive oil in a pan, add the chicken and cook for 6 minutes on each side. Serve with mixed salad leaves.

Ham & Egg Salad

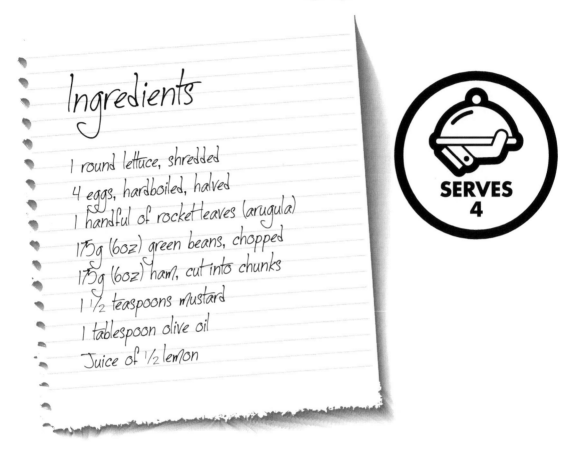

Ingredients

1 round lettuce, shredded
4 eggs, hardboiled, halved
1 handful of rocket leaves (arugula)
175g (6oz) green beans, chopped
175g (6oz) ham, cut into chunks
1 ½ teaspoons mustard
1 tablespoon olive oil
Juice of ½ lemon

SERVES
4

Method

Place the lemon juice, mustard and olive oil into a bowl and stir. Toss the rocket (arugula), lettuce, green beans, eggs and ham into the bowl and coat well with the dressing before serving.

Chicken & Vegetable Soup

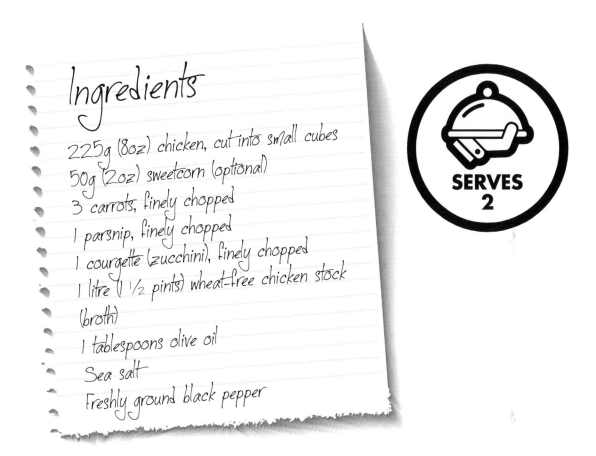

Ingredients

225g (8oz) chicken, cut into small cubes

50g (2oz) sweetcorn (optional)

3 carrots, finely chopped

1 parsnip, finely chopped

1 courgette (zucchini), finely chopped

1 litre (1 ½ pints) wheat-free chicken stock (broth)

1 tablespoons olive oil

Sea salt

Freshly ground black pepper

SERVES 2

Method

Heat the olive oil in a saucepan. Add the chicken and cook for 10 minutes. Add the courgette (zucchini), carrot and parsnip. Stir in the stock (broth). Continue cooking for around 20 minutes, until the vegetables are soft. Stir in the sweetcorn if you are using and warm through. Season the soup with salt and pepper and serve.

Pumpkin Soup

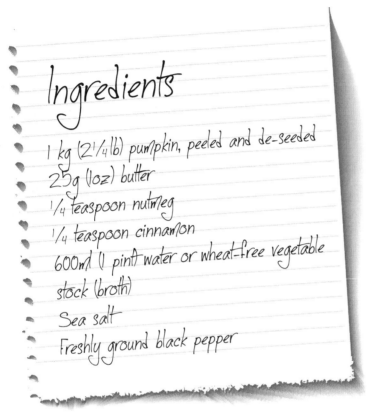

Ingredients

1 kg (2¼ lb) pumpkin, peeled and de-seeded
25g (1oz) butter
¼ teaspoon nutmeg
¼ teaspoon cinnamon
600ml (1 pint) water or wheat-free vegetable stock (broth)
Sea salt
Freshly ground black pepper

SERVES
6-8

Method

Cut the pumpkin flesh into cubes. Heat the butter in a saucepan, add the pumpkin and cook for 4 minutes. Add the water or stock (broth). Bring to the boil, reduce the heat and simmer for 30 minutes. Transfer to a food processor or use a hand blender to make a puree from the soup. Return to the pan and add the nutmeg, cinnamon, salt and pepper. Stir in some extra water or stock if you want it smoother. Serve and enjoy.

Thai Noodle Soup

Ingredients

400g (14oz) rice noodles
200g (7oz) pork mince
150g (5oz) bean sprouts
1 spring onion (scallion) green part only
finely chopped
450mls (15fl oz) wheat-free chicken stock
(broth)
300mls (10fl oz) water
2 teaspoons coriander leaves (cilantro),
chopped
1/2 teaspoon ground ginger

**SERVES
4**

Method

Heat the water and cook the noodles according to the instructions on the packet. In a bowl, combine the pork and ginger and form it into small balls of around 2cm (inch) in diameter. Bring the chicken stock (broth) to the boil, add the pork balls and boil for 7-8 minutes. Add the bean sprouts, coriander and spring onion (scallion) and cook for 3 minutes. Season and serve into bowls.

Gammon & Pineapple Salsa

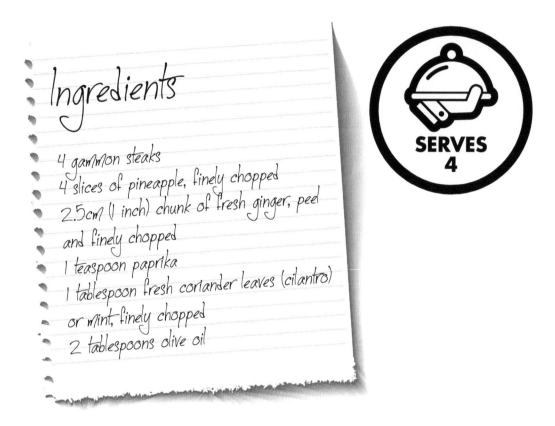

Ingredients

4 gammon steaks
4 slices of pineapple, finely chopped
2.5cm (1 inch) chunk of fresh ginger, peel and finely chopped
1 teaspoon paprika
1 tablespoon fresh coriander leaves (cilantro) or mint, finely chopped
2 tablespoons olive oil

SERVES 4

Method

Place the pineapple, ginger, paprika and coriander (cilantro) into a bowl with 1 tablespoon of olive oil and mix together. Make several incisions in the gammon fat to prevent it curling up during cooking. Heat a tablespoon olive oil in a frying pan, add the gammon steaks and cook for 5-6 minutes on each side until slightly golden. Serve with the pineapple salsa on the side.

Tuna & Broccoli Pasta

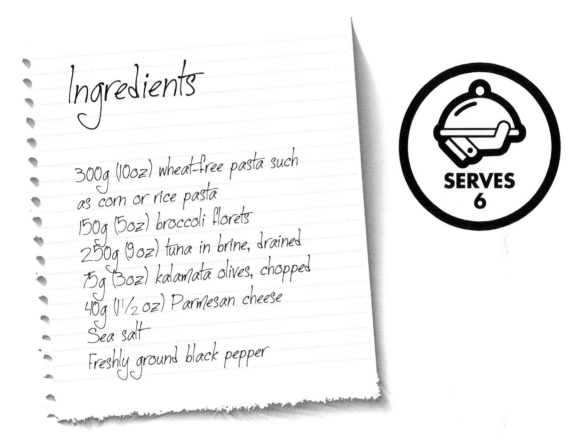

Ingredients

300g (10oz) wheat-free pasta such as corn or rice pasta
150g (5oz) broccoli florets
250g (9oz) tuna in brine, drained
75g (3oz) kalamata olives, chopped
40g (1½ oz) Parmesan cheese
Sea salt
Freshly ground black pepper

SERVES 6

Method

Cook the pasta according to the instructions. Steam the broccoli for 5-6 minutes until tender. Combine the broccoli with the pasta then add in the tuna, olives and sprinkle in the parmesan. Season with salt and pepper and serve.

Sicilian Pasta

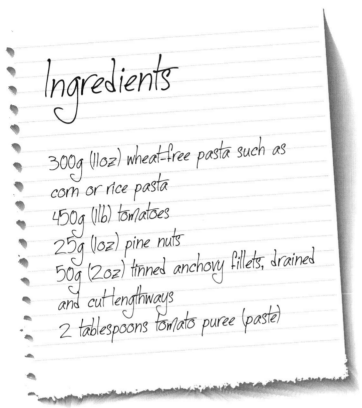

Ingredients

300g (11oz) wheat-free pasta such as corn or rice pasta

450g (1lb) tomatoes

25g (1oz) pine nuts

50g (2oz) tinned anchovy fillets, drained and cut lengthways

2 tablespoons tomato puree (paste)

SERVES
4

Method

Place the tomatoes under a hot grill (broiler) and cook for 8-10 minutes, turning occasionally. Place them in a bowl and cover with plastic film and allow to cool slightly. Remove the skin from the tomatoes and roughly chop the flesh. Dry fry the pine nuts for 1 minute until golden. Place the tomatoes and pine nuts into a saucepan and bring to the boil. Add the anchovies and tomato puree. Cook the wheat-free pasta according to the instructions then drain it. Combine the pasta with the sauce. Serve and eat immediately.

Salmon Burgers

Ingredients

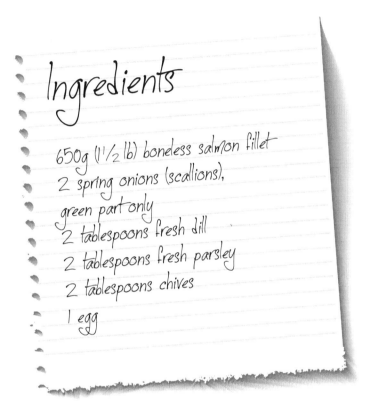

650g (1½ lb) boneless salmon fillet

2 spring onions (scallions), green part only

2 tablespoons fresh dill

2 tablespoons fresh parsley

2 tablespoons chives

1 egg

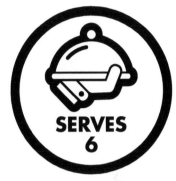

SERVES 6

Method

Put the salmon, spring onion (scallion), dill, parsley and chives into a food processor. Blend until smooth. Place the mixture in a medium bowl and combine with the egg. Shape the mixture into patties. Cook under a hot grill (broiler) for 15 minutes, turning once halfway through. Serve with mixed salad.

Tuna & Cheese Wraps

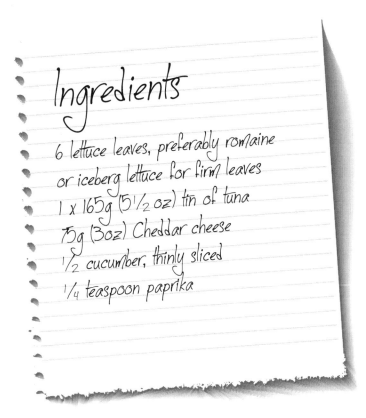

Ingredients

6 lettuce leaves, preferably romaine
or iceberg lettuce for firm leaves
1 x 165g (5½ oz) tin of tuna
75g (3oz) Cheddar cheese
½ cucumber, thinly sliced
¼ teaspoon paprika

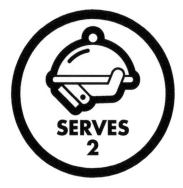

SERVES
2

Method

Combine the tuna, cheese and paprika in a bowl. Take a lettuce leaf and line it with
cucumber slices and top it off with a scoop of the tuna mixture. Eat straight away.
The combinations you can use for lettuce wraps are endless. You could try bacon,
tomato, olives, feta cheese, bean sprouts, leftover chicken or beef for a deliciously
light but filling lunch.

Almond & Lemon Baked Cod

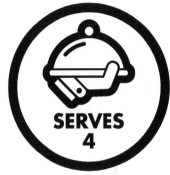

SERVES 4

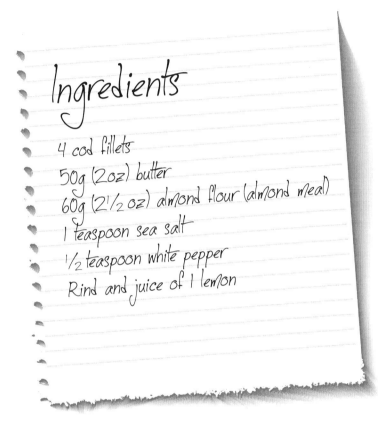

Ingredients

4 cod fillets
50g (2oz) butter
60g (2½ oz) almond flour (almond meal)
1 teaspoon sea salt
½ teaspoon white pepper
Rind and juice of 1 lemon

Method

Melt the butter in a saucepan and add the lemon juice and rind then set aside. On a plate, combine together the almond flour, salt and pepper. Dip the cod fillets into the lemon butter mixture then dip them into the almond flour making sure they are well coated. Lay out the fish on a baking tray. Bake in the oven at 180C/350F for around 25 minutes, or until the fish is flaky. Serve with a wedge of lemon.

Prawn & Red Pepper Kebabs

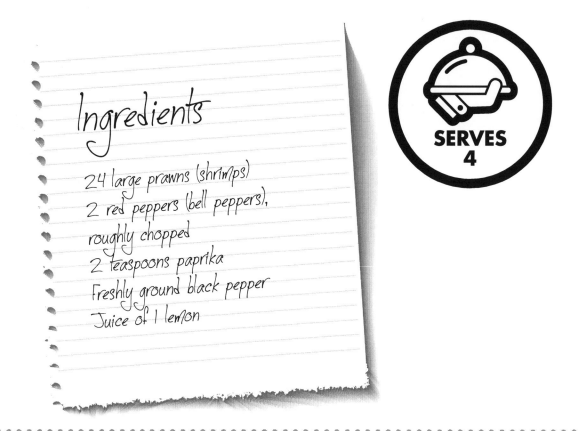

SERVES 4

Ingredients

24 large prawns (shrimps)
2 red peppers (bell peppers),
roughly chopped
2 teaspoons paprika
Freshly ground black pepper
Juice of 1 lemon

Method

Place the red peppers (bell peppers), prawns, lemon juice, paprika and black pepper into a bowl. Mix well. Slide alternating pieces of red pepper and prawns onto skewers. Place the kebabs under a hot grill (broiler) or a barbecue and cook for 3-4 minutes on each side, until cooked through.

Chilli & Tomato Prawns

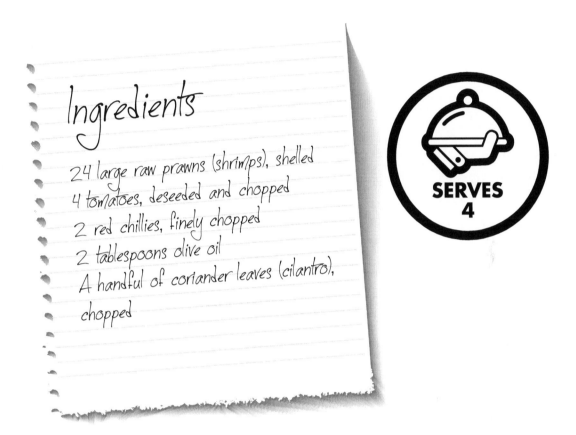

Ingredients

24 large raw prawns (shrimps), shelled
4 tomatoes, deseeded and chopped
2 red chillies, finely chopped
2 tablespoons olive oil
A handful of coriander leaves (cilantro), chopped

SERVES 4

Method

Heat a tablespoon of oil in a frying pan, add the prawns (shrimps) and cook until they are completely pink. Remove and set aside. Heat another tablespoon of oil in a pan and add the tomatoes and chilli peppers. Cook for 3 minutes. Return the prawns to the pan and warm through. Sprinkle with chopped coriander (cilantro) and stir. Serve with rice and salad.

Lemony Herb Quinoa Salad

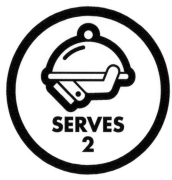

SERVES 2

Ingredients

250g (9oz) quinoa, cooked

1/2 cucumber, peeled and diced

6 cherry tomatoes, quartered

2 tablespoons fresh basil, finely chopped

2 tablespoons fresh coriander, (cilantro), finely chopped

2 tablespoons fresh parsley, finely chopped

6 pitted olives, finely chopped

60ml (2fl oz) olive oil

Juice of 2 lemons

Sea salt

Freshly ground black pepper

Method

In a large bowl, mix together the, olive oil, lemon juice, salt, and pepper. Add the quinoa, tomatoes, cucumber, olives, and herbs. Toss all of the ingredients in the dressing until they are thoroughly coated. Chill in the fridge for 1 hour before serving.

Bacon & Swede Hash

Ingredients

4 carrots, peeled and chopped
1 small swede, peeled and chopped
6 slices of bacon, roughly chopped
1 tablespoon olive oil
Pinch of nutmeg (optional)
Sea salt
Freshly ground black pepper

SERVES 4

Method

Steam the carrot and swede until tender. Drain off the water, mash it and add the nutmeg if using. Heat the olive oil in a frying pan. Add the bacon and fry until it's cooked. Add the carrot and swede to the pan and stir. Cook for around 5 minutes until it becomes crispy at the bottom of the pan. Serve and eat straight away. This recipe also works well with leftover vegetables.

Mozzarella Potato Skins

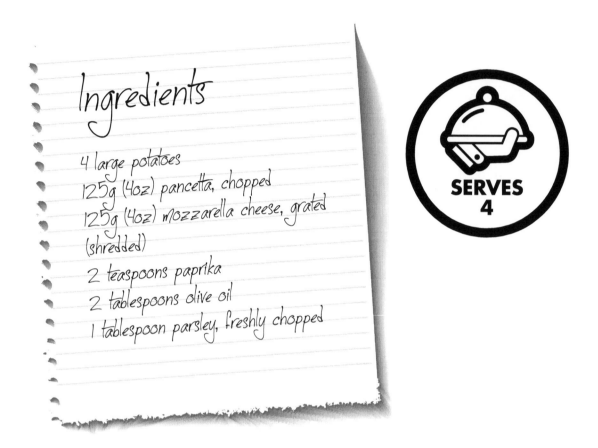

Ingredients

4 large potatoes
125g (4oz) pancetta, chopped
125g (4oz) mozzarella cheese, grated (shredded)
2 teaspoons paprika
2 tablespoons olive oil
1 tablespoon parsley, freshly chopped

SERVES 4

Method

Preheat the oven to 200C/400F. Prick potatoes with a fork and place them on the top shelf of the oven. Bake for 1 hour or until soft in the middle and leave to cool. Cut the potatoes in half, scoop the flesh into a bowl and set aside. Combine the oil and paprika and use some of it to brush the outside of the potato skins. Place under a hot grill for 5 minutes, until crisp, turning occasionally. Heat the remaining oil and paprika and fry the pancetta until it's crispy. Add this to the potato flesh, along with the mozzarella and parsley. Mix well. Fill the potato skins with the mixture. Place the skins in the oven for a further 15 minutes until heated thoroughly.

Ham & Pepper Pizza

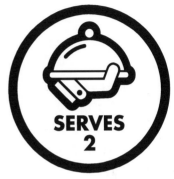

SERVES 2

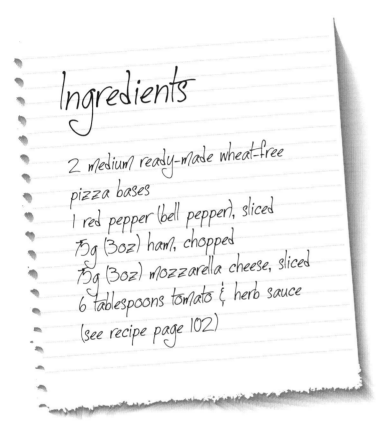

Ingredients

2 medium ready-made wheat-free pizza bases

1 red pepper (bell pepper), sliced

75g (3oz) ham, chopped

75g (3oz) mozzarella cheese, sliced

6 tablespoons tomato & herb sauce (see recipe page 102)

Method

Spread the tomato sauce over the pizza bases and sprinkle the cheese, red pepper and ham on top. Bake for 15 minutes until the cheese has melted. Serve and eat immediately. Alternatively try different toppings like feta, prawns, bacon, courgette, olives, spinach, tomatoes, chicken, beef, pork, chives, basil and oregano.

Tomato & Aubergine (Eggplant) Gratin

SERVES 4-6

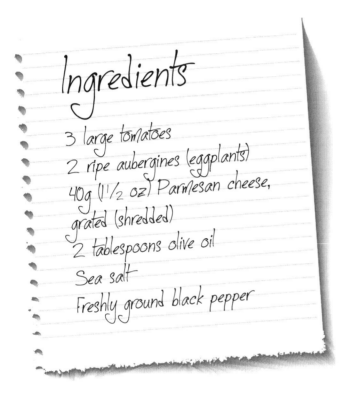

Ingredients

3 large tomatoes
2 ripe aubergines (eggplants)
40g (1½ oz) Parmesan cheese, grated (shredded)
2 tablespoons olive oil
Sea salt
Freshly ground black pepper

Method

Cut the tomatoes into slices and set aside. Thinly slice the aubergines (eggplants) and place them on a grill rack lined with foil. Brush with olive oil and grill (broil) for 15 minutes, turning once until golden on both sides. Place the tomato slices and aubergine slices in an oven-proof dish, alternating between slices of each. Cover with the grated Parmesan and season with salt and pepper. Transfer to the oven and bake at 200C/400F for 15 minutes, or until the cheese is golden. Serve and eat immediately.

DINNER

Creamy Chicken Curry

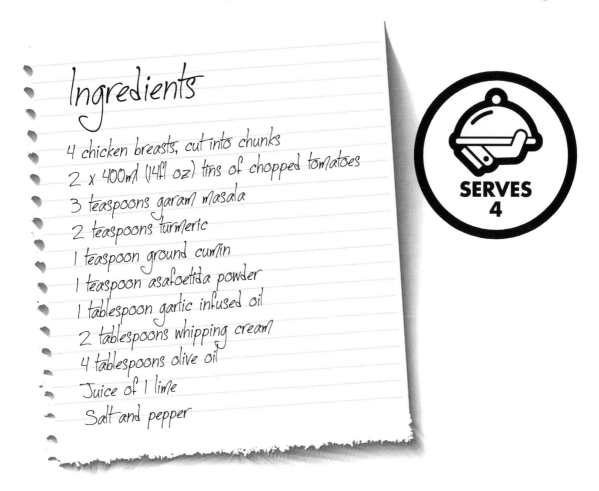

Ingredients

4 chicken breasts, cut into chunks
2 x 400ml (14fl oz) tins of chopped tomatoes
3 teaspoons garam masala
2 teaspoons turmeric
1 teaspoon ground cumin
1 teaspoon asafoetida powder
1 tablespoon garlic infused oil
2 tablespoons whipping cream
4 tablespoons olive oil
Juice of 1 lime
Salt and pepper

SERVES 4

Method

Marinate the chicken with the lime juice and a sprinkling of salt. In the meantime, heat 3 tablespoons of oil in a pan. Add the garam masala, turmeric, asafoetida and cumin. Stir and cook for 2 minutes. Add in the tinned tomatoes, garlic infused oil and season with salt and pepper. Bring to the boil, reduce the heat and simmer for 20 minutes. In a separate saucepan, heat a tablespoon of olive oil and brown the chicken for 5 minutes. Once the curry sauce has cooled slightly use a hand blender or food processor and blitz until smooth. Return it to the heat, add in the chicken and simmer for 15-20 minutes. Stir in the cream and serve with rice.

Chicken Satay

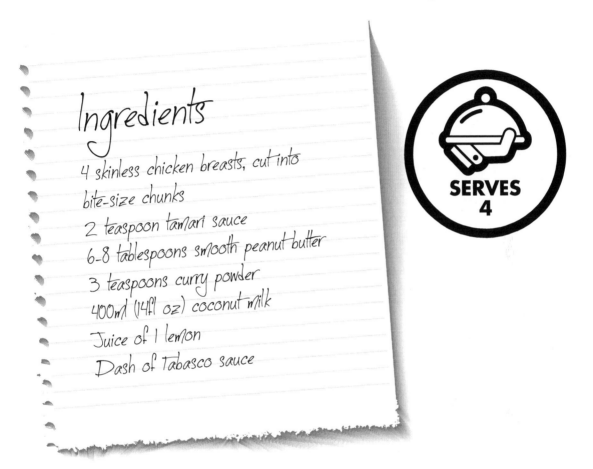

Ingredients

4 skinless chicken breasts, cut into bite-size chunks

2 teaspoon tamari sauce

6-8 tablespoons smooth peanut butter

3 teaspoons curry powder

400ml (14fl oz) coconut milk

Juice of 1 lemon

Dash of Tabasco sauce

SERVES 4

Method

Preheat the oven to 200C/400F. In a bowl, combine the peanut butter and coconut milk. Stir in the curry powder, Tabasco and tamari sauce. Thoroughly coat the chicken chunks in the peanut mixture. Thread the chicken onto skewers, and set aside the remaining satay sauce. Place the chicken skewers under a hot grill (broiler) and cook for 4-5 minutes on each side, making sure they are thoroughly cooked. Pour the remaining satay sauce into a small saucepan and add the juice from half of the lemon and bring to the boil. Serve the chicken skewers and pour the remaining satay sauce on top.

Parsnip & Potato Bake

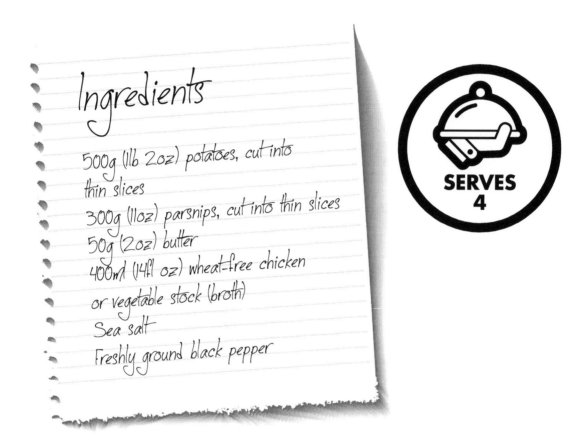

Ingredients

500g (1lb 2oz) potatoes, cut into thin slices

300g (11oz) parsnips, cut into thin slices

50g (2oz) butter

400ml (14fl oz) wheat-free chicken or vegetable stock (broth)

Sea salt

Freshly ground black pepper

SERVES 4

Method

Butter a casserole dish and arrange the sliced parsnip and potatoes into layers. Season with salt and pepper. Pour in enough stock (broth) to cover the vegetable slices. Flake pieces of butter over the dish. Transfer to the oven and bake at 180C/360F for about 35 minutes until slightly golden on top. Serve as an accompaniment to meat and fish dishes.

Mixed Vegetable Casserole

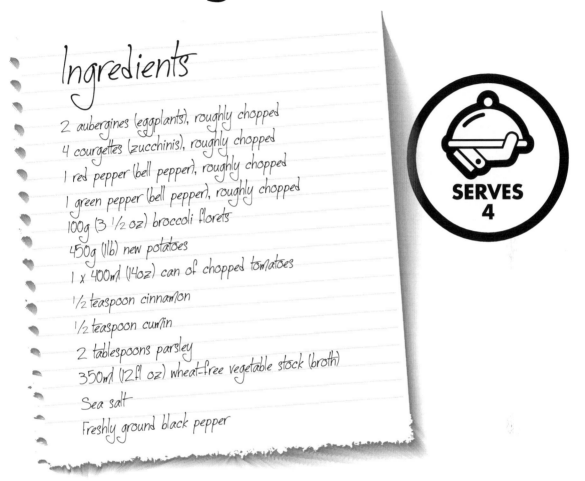

Ingredients

2 aubergines (eggplants), roughly chopped

4 courgettes (zucchinis), roughly chopped

1 red pepper (bell pepper), roughly chopped

1 green pepper (bell pepper), roughly chopped

100g (3 ½ oz) broccoli florets

450g (1lb) new potatoes

1 x 400ml (14oz) can of chopped tomatoes

½ teaspoon cinnamon

½ teaspoon cumin

2 tablespoons parsley

350ml (12fl oz) wheat-free vegetable stock (broth)

Sea salt

Freshly ground black pepper

SERVES 4

Method

Heat the olive oil in a frying pan. Add the potatoes, broccoli, aubergines (eggplants), courgettes (zucchinis) peppers, spices and salt and pepper. Cook for 5 minutes. Transfer the ingredients to an ovenproof casserole dish. Pour on the tomatoes, vegetable stock (broth) and season with salt and pepper. Place in the oven at 190C/375F for 40 minutes. Stir in the parsley and serve.

Slow Cooked Lamb

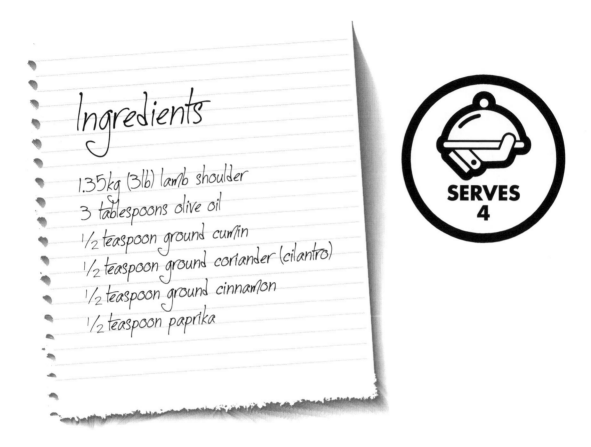

Ingredients

1.35kg (3lb) lamb shoulder
3 tablespoons olive oil
1/2 teaspoon ground cumin
1/2 teaspoon ground coriander (cilantro)
1/2 teaspoon ground cinnamon
1/2 teaspoon paprika

SERVES 4

Method

Mix the spices with a tablespoon of olive oil. Coat the lamb with the mixture and marinate it for an hour, or longer if you can. Heat the remaining oil in a pan, add the lamb and brown it for 3-4 minutes on all sides to seal it. Place the lamb in an ovenproof dish and cover it with foil. Transfer to the oven and roast at 170C/325F for 4 hours. The lamb should be tender and falling off the bone. Shred the lamb and serve onto a dish. This is an excellent meal for sharing. Serve with quinoa and vegetables.

Almond Crusted Chicken Goujons

Ingredients

4 chicken breasts, cut into strips

75g (3oz) ground almonds (almond meal)

1 egg

1/2 teaspoon white pepper

1/2 teaspoon paprika

2 tablespoons butter

1/4 teaspoon salt

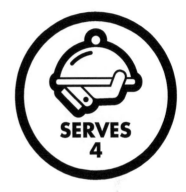

SERVES 4

Method

Place the ground almonds into a bowl with the paprika, salt and pepper and mix well. In a separate bowl, beat the egg. Dip the chicken strips into the egg, then dip it into the almond mixture and coat thoroughly. Heat the butter in a frying pan and add the chicken. Cook for about 5-6 minutes on each side until the chicken is golden and cooked thoroughly.

Pumpkin Risotto

Ingredients

SERVES 6

50g (2oz) butter
900g (2lb) pumpkin, peeled, de-seeded and cubed
225g (8oz) risotto rice (Arborio)
600ml (1 pint) wheat-free chicken stock (broth)
40g (1 1/2oz) Parmesan cheese, grated
2 tablespoons chives, chopped
Sea salt
Freshly ground black pepper

Method

Melt the butter in a saucepan. Add the pumpkin and fry until soft. Add the rice then mix well. Add in the stock (broth) a little at a time. Allow the rice to absorb most of the liquid before you add more. It will take around 20-25 minutes. Season it with salt and pepper. Sprinkle with Parmesan and chives stir. Serve and enjoy.

Chive & Potato Cakes

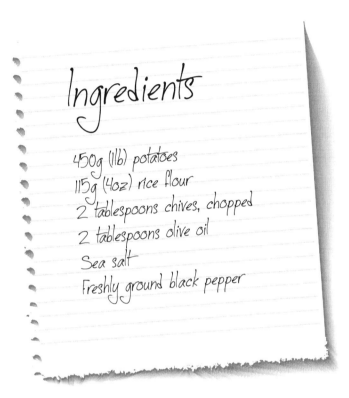

Ingredients

450g (1lb) potatoes
115g (4oz) rice flour
2 tablespoons chives, chopped
2 tablespoons olive oil
Sea salt
Freshly ground black pepper

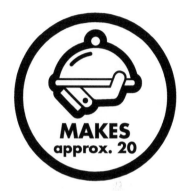

MAKES
approx. 20

Method

Boil the potatoes in salted water for 20 minutes before draining and mashing them. Season with salt and pepper. Add the rice flour, chives and olive oil and mix well until you have a soft dough. Roll out the mixture onto a floured surface. To a depth of ½ cm (¼ inch). Using a pastry cutter cut small rounds of around 5cm (2 inches). Heat a lightly greased frying pan and cook the cakes for around 10 minutes until golden brown, turning once. Serve hot and top with a little butter. These go really well with bacon and eggs.

Cottage Pie

Ingredients

800g (1 ³/₄ lb) potatoes, peeled and chopped into small cubes

125g (4oz) streaky bacon, chopped

450g (1lb) minced beef (ground beef)

50g (2oz) Cheddar cheese, grated (shredded)

1 courgette (zucchini), chopped

400ml (14fl oz) wheat-free beef or vegetable stock (broth)

1 tablespoon fresh parsley, chopped

3 tablespoons fresh chives, chopped

2 tablespoons tomato puree (paste)

3 tablespoons butter

Sea salt

Freshly ground black pepper

SERVES 4-6

Method

In a large pan, fry the bacon until cooked and set aside. Add the beef to the pan and cook for 2 minutes. Add the stock (broth), courgette (zucchini), tomato puree (paste), parsley and chives. Season with salt and pepper. Cover and cook for 30 minutes, stirring occasionally. In the meantime, boil the potatoes until tender. Drain the potatoes, add the butter and mash them. Preheat the oven to 200C/400F. Place the beef mixture in the bottom of an ovenproof casserole dish. Add the mashed potato layer on top and smooth it out with the back of a spoon. Sprinkle with cheese and bake in the oven for around 20 minutes or until the pie is lightly browned and the cheese melted.

Saffron Roast Chicken

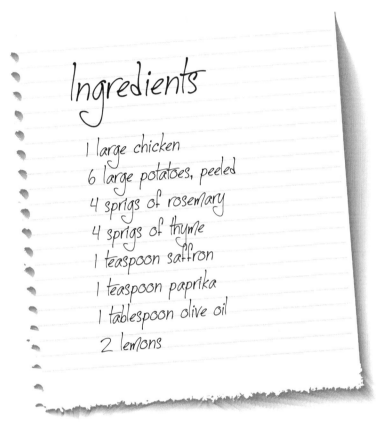

Ingredients

1 large chicken
6 large potatoes, peeled
4 sprigs of rosemary
4 sprigs of thyme
1 teaspoon saffron
1 teaspoon paprika
1 tablespoon olive oil
2 lemons

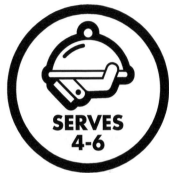

SERVES 4-6

Method

Cut one of the lemons into quarters and insert into the cavity of the chicken. Make some incisions in the skin and insert the sprigs of herbs. Sprinkle the saffron over the chicken. Slice the remaining lemon and place the pieces on top of the saffron to stop it from drying out. Put the chicken into an ovenproof dish or baking tray. Quarter the potatoes, place them in the tray and coat them with oil and paprika. Place in the oven at 180C/360F for around 1 hour 20 minutes. Adjust the cooking time depending on the size of the chicken. Test with a skewer for the juices to run clear before removing.

Herby Monkfish Skewers

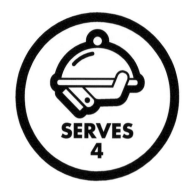

SERVES 4

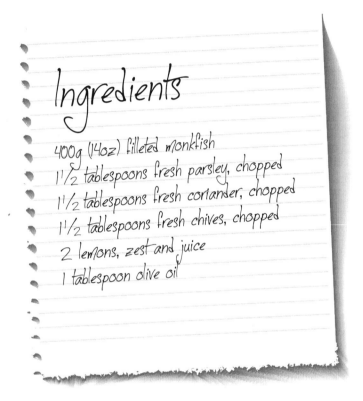

Ingredients

400g (14oz) filleted monkfish

1½ tablespoons fresh parsley, chopped

1½ tablespoons fresh coriander, chopped

1½ tablespoons fresh chives, chopped

2 lemons, zest and juice

1 tablespoon olive oil

Method

Cut the monkfish into bite-size chunks. Combine the lemon juice, zest, herbs and oil in a bowl or alternatively place it in blender and blitz until smooth. Coat the monkfish in the marinade and thread on skewers. Place the skewers on a barbecue or under a grill (broiler) and cook for around 3 minutes on each side until cooked thoroughly. Serve with rice and salad.

Lemon Chicken

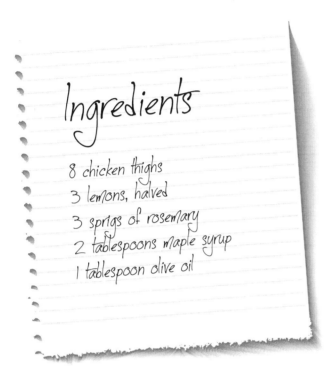

Ingredients

8 chicken thighs
3 lemons, halved
3 sprigs of rosemary
2 tablespoons maple syrup
1 tablespoon olive oil

SERVES
4

Method

Combine the maple syrup, olive oil and juice from the lemons in a casserole dish.
Add the chicken thighs and coat them in the mixture. Stuff the squeezed lemon halves
around the chicken. Break the sprigs of rosemary in half and add them to the dish.
Transfer to the oven and bake at 180C/360F for 1 hour.

Beef Kebabs

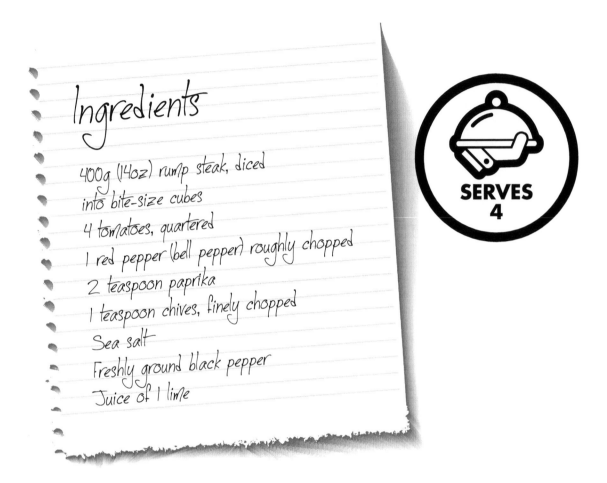

Ingredients

400g (14oz) rump steak, diced into bite-size cubes

4 tomatoes, quartered

1 red pepper (bell pepper) roughly chopped

2 teaspoon paprika

1 teaspoon chives, finely chopped

Sea salt

Freshly ground black pepper

Juice of 1 lime

SERVES 4

Method

Mix together the paprika, lime juice, chives, salt and pepper in a bowl. Add the steak cubes, tomatoes and red pepper (bell pepper). Stir to coat the ingredients with the mixture. Thread the steak and vegetables onto skewers, alternating them as you go. Place under a preheated grill for 9-10 minutes turning during cooking ensure they're evenly cooked.

Chicken & Red Pepper Risotto

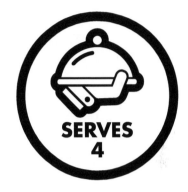

SERVES 4

Ingredients

300g (11oz) risotto rice (Arborio)

1200ml (2 pints) warm wheat-free chicken stock (broth)

100g (3½oz) spinach

125g (4oz) cooked chicken, chopped

1 red pepper (bell pepper), chopped

1 tablespoon olive oil

Salt & black pepper

Method

Heat the olive oil in and a saucepan. Add the red pepper (bell pepper) and cook for around 5 minutes until softened. Add the rice to the pan, stir and cook for 2 minutes, until the rice is coated in oil. Slowly add the stock (broth) while stirring and adding a little at a time until all the liquid has been absorbed, around 20 minutes. Add the spinach and chicken to the pan. Cook until the spinach has wilted – around 2 minutes. Season and serve.

Aubergine and Feta Towers

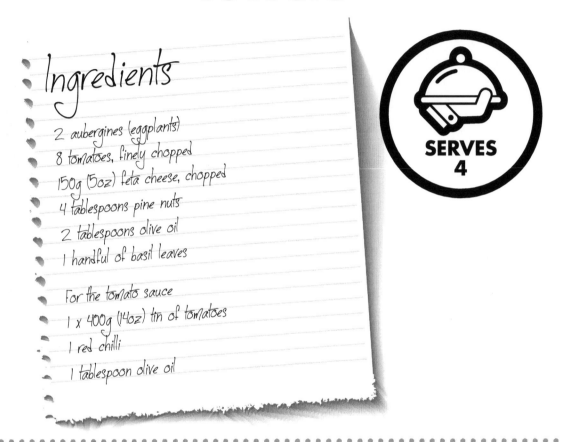

SERVES 4

Ingredients

2 aubergines (eggplants)

8 tomatoes, finely chopped

150g (5oz) feta cheese, chopped

4 tablespoons pine nuts

2 tablespoons olive oil

1 handful of basil leaves

For the tomato sauce

1 x 400g (14oz) tin of tomatoes

1 red chilli

1 tablespoon olive oil

Method

Cut the aubergines (eggplants) into slices of around 2.5cm (1 inch) thick. Heat 2 tablespoons of oil in a pan, add the aubergine and cook for 3 minutes on either side. Remove and set aside. In a bowl, combine the tomatoes, basil and feta cheese. Dry fry the pine nuts for 1 minute until lightly toasted and mix them with the tomatoes and cheese. On a baking sheet, place the 4 largest slices of aubergine and add a spoonful of the tomato mixture. Select the next largest pieces, place on top, followed by more tomato mixture. Continue like this until you have 4 slices of aubergine stacked on top of each other with the tomato mixture in between. Transfer to the oven and cook at 180/360F for 12 minutes. In the meantime, place the tomatoes, chilli and olive oil into a blender and blitz until smooth then heat it in a saucepan. Serve the aubergine towers and spoon the tomato sauce onto the side.

Mediterranean Style Cod

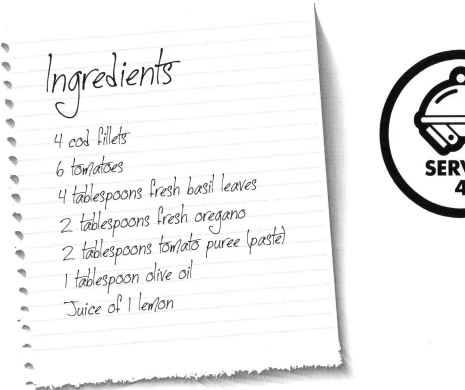

Ingredients

4 cod fillets
6 tomatoes
4 tablespoons fresh basil leaves
2 tablespoons fresh oregano
2 tablespoons tomato puree (paste)
1 tablespoon olive oil
Juice of 1 lemon

SERVES 4

Method

Place the tomatoes, lemon juice, olive oil, basil, oregano and tomato puree (paste) into a blender and process until mixed but not yet too smooth. Place the cod fillets on a baking tray and cover them with the tomato mixture. Place them in the oven at 180C/360F for 18 minutes.

Turkey Curry

Ingredients

4 turkey steaks, cut into strips
1 large red pepper (bell pepper)
400ml (14fl oz) coconut milk
2 teaspoon ground ginger
2 tablespoons curry powder
1 tablespoons ground turmeric
1 tablespoons ground coriander (cilantro)
1 teaspoon ground turmeric
3 tablespoons olive oil
Juice of 1 lime
Small bunch of fresh coriander (cilantro) leaves, chopped

SERVES 4

Method

Heat the olive oil in a saucepan and add the turkey strips. Cook for 5 minutes then transfer to a plate and keep warm. Place the spices into the saucepan together with the red pepper (bell pepper). Stir and cook for around 2 minutes. Pour in the coconut milk and add the lime juice. Bring to the boil, reduce the heat. Add the turkey to the saucepan and simmer for 15 minutes. Sprinkle in the coriander (cilantro) and stir. Serve with rice.

Ginger & Balsamic Steaks

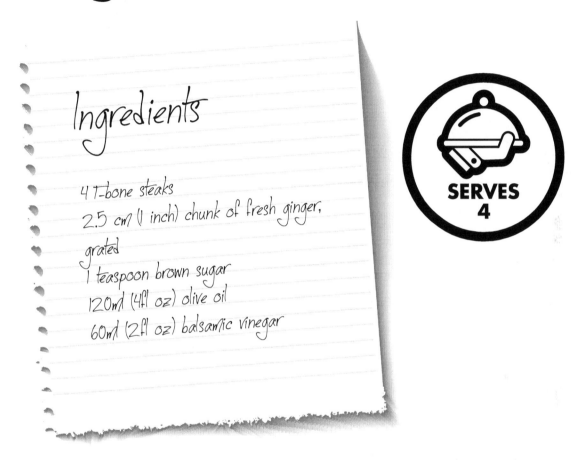

Ingredients

4 T-bone steaks
2.5 cm (1 inch) chunk of fresh ginger, grated
1 teaspoon brown sugar
120ml (4fl oz) olive oil
60ml (2fl oz) balsamic vinegar

SERVES 4

Method

Mix together the vinegar, oil, sugar and ginger. Place half of the mixture into a separate container and marinate the steaks in the remaining oil and vinegar for several minutes. Place the steaks under a hot grill and cook on each side until done the way you like it, basting occasionally with the oil/vinegar mixture. Serve onto a bed of green salad and pour over the vinegar mixture you had reserved.

Sweet & Sour Pork

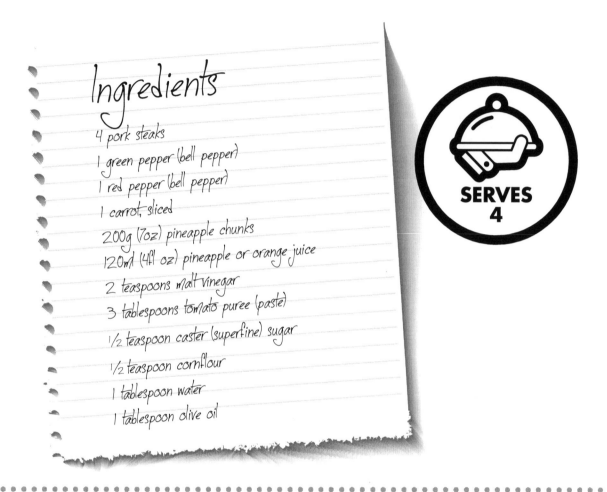

Ingredients

- 4 pork steaks
- 1 green pepper (bell pepper)
- 1 red pepper (bell pepper)
- 1 carrot, sliced
- 200g (7oz) pineapple chunks
- 120ml (4fl oz) pineapple or orange juice
- 2 teaspoons malt vinegar
- 3 tablespoons tomato puree (paste)
- 1/2 teaspoon caster (superfine) sugar
- 1/2 teaspoon cornflour
- 1 tablespoon water
- 1 tablespoon olive oil

SERVES 4

Method

Grill the pork steaks for 5 minutes on each side and allow them to cool then cut into bite-size chunks. Heat the oil in a frying pan and add the peppers (bell peppers) and carrot. Cook for 1 minute. Add the pineapple chunks, juice, vinegar, tomato puree, and sugar. Cook for 3 minutes. Add in the pork and cook for 2 minutes. In a cup, mix together the cornflour and water to make a smooth paste. Stir it into the pan and mix until thickened. Serve with rice.

Pesto Lamb Chops

Ingredients

8 lamb chops
1 tablespoon olive oil
Salt & pepper

For the pesto
4 tablespoons pine nuts
6 tablespoons basil leaves
75g (3oz) Parmesan cheese, finely grated
2 tablespoons olive oil

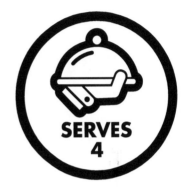

SERVES 4

Method

For the pesto: put all of the ingredients into a blender and blitz until you have a smooth paste. Set it aside. Season the chops with salt and pepper. Heat the oil in a pan and fry them for 2-3 minutes on each side, or longer if you like them well done. Transfer to a plate and cover with pesto. Serve alongside a green salad and new potatoes.

Prosciutto Wrapped Prawns (Shrimps)

SERVES 4

Ingredients

20 large peeled, deveined, prawns (shrimps)
10 slices prosciutto
1 tablespoon fresh basil, chopped
1/2 teaspoon lemon zest
1/2 teaspoon sea salt
1/2 teaspoon chilli flakes
Pinch of freshly ground black pepper
1 lemon, quartered for garnish
1 teaspoon olive oil

Method

In a medium bowl, combine the prawns (shrimps), basil, olive oil, lemon zest, salt, chilli flakes and black pepper. Mix well and set aside. Lay out the prosciutto in slices, and cut it in half lengthwise so you have 20 pieces. Wrap the prosciutto around each shrimp then thread onto a skewer. Repeat for the remaining prawns and place 5 prawns on each skewer. Place the skewers under a grill (broiler) and cook for around 2 minutes on each side. Serve hot with lemon wedges.

Spare Ribs

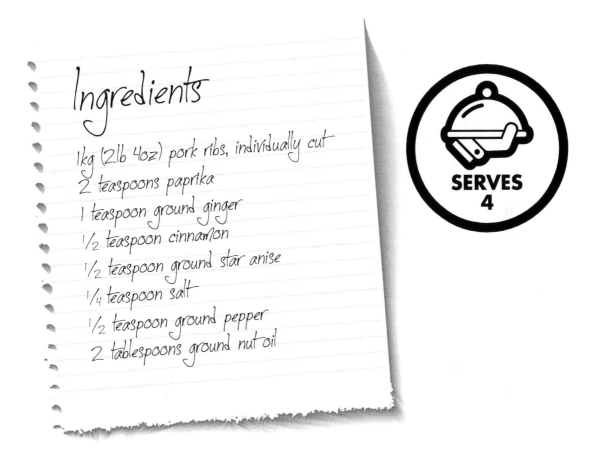

Ingredients

1kg (2lb 4oz) pork ribs, individually cut
2 teaspoons paprika
1 teaspoon ground ginger
1/2 teaspoon cinnamon
1/2 teaspoon ground star anise
1/4 teaspoon salt
1/2 teaspoon ground pepper
2 tablespoons ground nut oil

SERVES 4

Method

Place the spices, salt, pepper and oil in a bowl and combine. Coat the ribs with the mixture making sure they're evenly coated. Place the pork ribs in a roasting tin and cook them in the oven at 180C/360F for 35-40 minutes. Alternatively the ribs can be cooked a barbecue once they've been coated. Place on a large serving plate and eat them while hot.

Pork Escalope
with Noodles

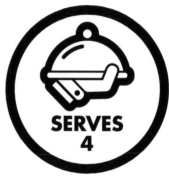

**SERVES
4**

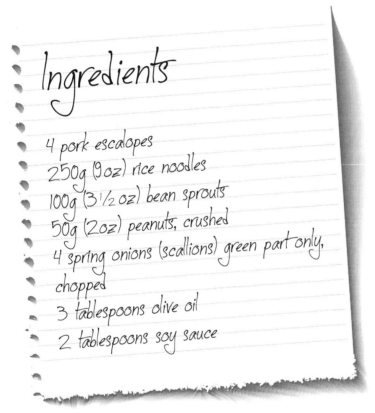

Ingredients

4 pork escalopes
250g (9oz) rice noodles
100g (3½ oz) bean sprouts
50g (2oz) peanuts, crushed
4 spring onions (scallions) green part only,
chopped
3 tablespoons olive oil
2 tablespoons soy sauce

Method

Heat a tablespoon olive oil in a pan and add the pork escalopes. Cook for 2-3 minutes on either side or until cook thoroughly. Cook the noodles according to their instructions. Remove the pork and keep warm. Place 2 tablespoons of olive oil in a pan add the soy sauce, bean sprouts, chopped spring onion, peanuts and warm through. Add the noodles and stir. Serve onto plates and add the pork escalope onto top.

Parmesan Chicken

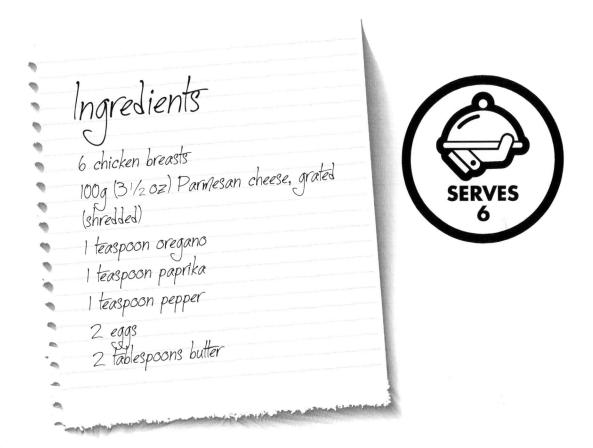

Ingredients

6 chicken breasts

100g (3½ oz) Parmesan cheese, grated (shredded)

1 teaspoon oregano

1 teaspoon paprika

1 teaspoon pepper

2 eggs

2 tablespoons butter

SERVES 6

Method

In a bowl, combine the Parmesan cheese with the oregano, paprika and pepper. In a separate bowl, whisk the eggs. Dip the chicken breasts in the beaten egg, followed by a generous dip in the cheese and herb mixture, making sure you coat both sides really well. Melt the butter in a frying pan over a medium heat. Add the chicken breasts and cook for 4 or 5 minutes on each side, or until cooked through.

Mustard & Ginger Chicken

Ingredients

4 chicken breasts
2.5cm (1 inch) chunk of root ginger, crushed
300ml (10fl oz) chicken stock (broth)
1 teaspoon Tabasco sauce
1 teaspoon paprika
2 teaspoons mustard
1 teaspoon sugar
Sea Salt
Freshly ground black pepper
1 tablespoon olive oil

Method

Heat the olive oil in a frying pan and add the chicken breasts. Cook the chicken for 4 minutes on each side or until golden then remove them, cover and set aside. Add the ginger to the pan and cook for 1 minute. Add the stock (broth), mustard, paprika, Tabasco sauce and sugar. Bring to the boil then reduce the heat. Return the chicken to the pan and simmer gently for 10 minutes. Season with salt and pepper before serving.

Barbecue Chicken Wings

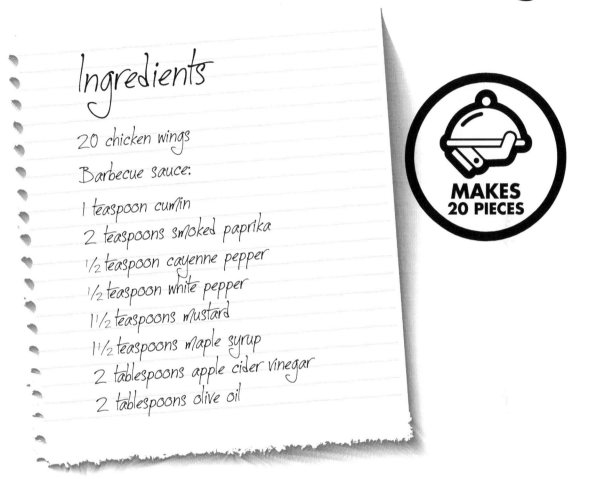

Ingredients

20 chicken wings

Barbecue sauce:

1 teaspoon cumin
2 teaspoons smoked paprika
½ teaspoon cayenne pepper
½ teaspoon white pepper
1½ teaspoons mustard
1½ teaspoons maple syrup
2 tablespoons apple cider vinegar
2 tablespoons olive oil

MAKES 20 PIECES

Method

Preheat the oven to 200C/400F. In a bowl, mix together all the barbecue sauce ingredients and stir really well. Coat the chicken wings in the sauce and place them on a large baking sheet. Transfer to the oven for 30 minutes, until the chicken is cooked through and golden brown. Serve with a green salad and enjoy.

Peanut & Sesame Chicken

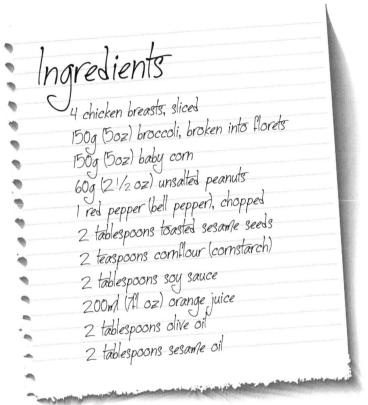

Ingredients

4 chicken breasts, sliced
150g (5oz) broccoli, broken into florets
150g (5oz) baby corn
60g (2½ oz) unsalted peanuts
1 red pepper (bell pepper), chopped
2 tablespoons toasted sesame seeds
2 teaspoons cornflour (cornstarch)
2 tablespoons soy sauce
200ml (7fl oz) orange juice
2 tablespoons olive oil
2 tablespoons sesame oil

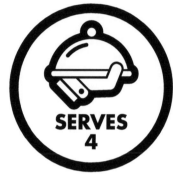

SERVES
4

Method

Heat both of the oils in a large frying pan. Add the chicken and cook for 4-5 minutes.
Add in the broccoli, red pepper (bell pepper) and baby corn. Stir and cook for 2 minutes.
In a separate bowl mix the soy sauce, orange juice and cornflour. Pour it into the pan
with the chicken and vegetables. The sauce will thicken and form a glaze. Sprinkle on the
peanuts and sesame seeds and warm them through. Serve with rice noodles or rice.

DESSERTS, SWEET TREATS & SNACKS

Coconut Macaroons

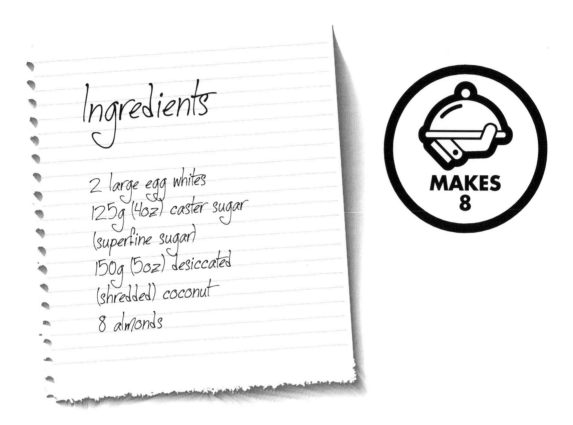

Ingredients

2 large egg whites
125g (4oz) caster sugar
(superfine sugar)
150g (5oz) desiccated
(shredded) coconut
8 almonds

MAKES
8

Method

Grease and line a baking sheet. Place the separated egg whites in a bowl and whisk into soft peaks. Add in the coconut and sugar using a metal spoon and fold until thoroughly mixed in. Spoon the mixture onto the baking sheet, making 8 large rounded shapes. Place an almond on top of each one. Transfer to the oven and bake at 180C/360F for 15-20 minutes until golden. Allow to cool for 5 minutes then transfer them to a wire rack.

Chocolate Ice Cream

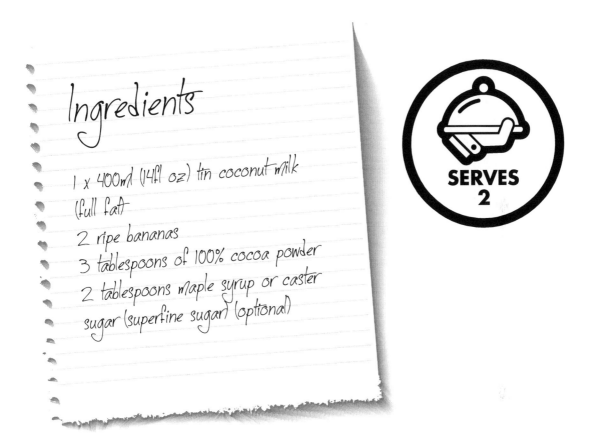

Ingredients

1 x 400ml (14fl oz) tin coconut milk (full fat

2 ripe bananas

3 tablespoons of 100% cocoa powder

2 tablespoons maple syrup or caster sugar (superfine sugar) (optional)

SERVES 2

Method

Place the bananas, coconut milk and cocoa powder into a blender. Blitz until smooth. The mixture is already fairly sweet, however taste it and add maple syrup or stevia if you wish to make it sweeter. Transfer it to an ice cream maker and process it for the required time depending on your machine. Freeze or eat straight away.

Crème Caramel

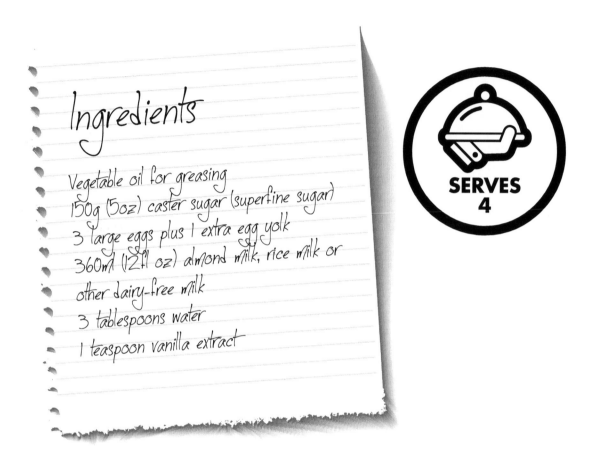

Ingredients

Vegetable oil for greasing
150g (5oz) caster sugar (superfine sugar)
3 large eggs plus 1 extra egg yolk
360ml (12fl oz) almond milk, rice milk or
other dairy-free milk
3 tablespoons water
1 teaspoon vanilla extract

SERVES 4

Method

Grease four ramekins with a little vegetable oil. Put 125g (4oz) sugar into a saucepan and add the 3 tablespoons of water. Heat gently for 6–8 minutes until the sugar has caramelised taking care not to burn it. Pour the caramel into the ramekins. Use a mixer to beat together the eggs, extra egg yolk and the vanilla extract with the remaining sugar. Mix it until thick and smooth. Pour the milk into a saucepan and bring to the boil. Remove from the heat and slowly add the milk to the egg mixture and mix thoroughly.

Divide the milk mixture into the individual ramekins and put them in a roasting dish. Pour enough boiling water into the roasting dish to come halfway up the sides of the ramekins. Bake at 150C/300F for 30–35 minutes until set firm and golden. Remove from the oven and leave to cool. Cover and leave to chill in the fridge for 10-12 hours. Serve chilled.

Banana Bread

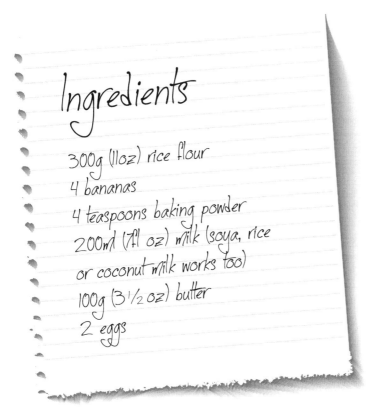

Ingredients

300g (11oz) rice flour
4 bananas
4 teaspoons baking powder
200ml (7fl oz) milk (soya, rice
or coconut milk works too)
100g (3½ oz) butter
2 eggs

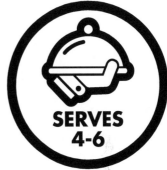

**SERVES
4-6**

Method

Place all the ingredients into a food processor and process until smooth. Line a large
loaf tin with greaseproof parchment paper. Spread the mixture into the tin. Heat the
oven to 180C/360F. Bake for 35 minutes. Check to see if it's done using a skewer
which should come out clean. Turn out of the tin and allow it to cool before serving.

Creamy Cinnamon Rice Pudding

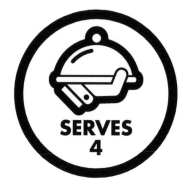

SERVES 4

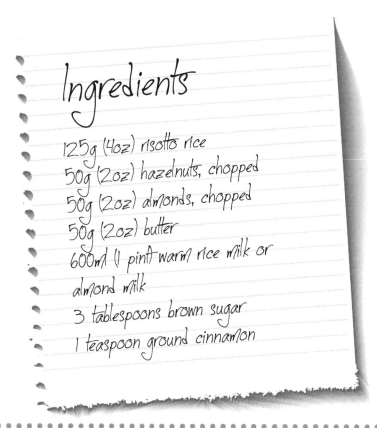

Ingredients

125g (4oz) risotto rice
50g (2oz) hazelnuts, chopped
50g (2oz) almonds, chopped
50g (2oz) butter
600ml (1 pint) warm rice milk or
almond milk
3 tablespoons brown sugar
1 teaspoon ground cinnamon

Method

Heat a frying pan, add the chopped nuts and toast until golden, then set aside. Heat the butter in a saucepan, stir in the rice and cook for around 1 minute. Slowly add the warm milk to the rice, stirring continuously. Add the sugar and cinnamon and simmer gently for around 20 minutes until the rice is soft. Serve the rice pudding into bowls and sprinkle with the toasted nuts.

Flapjacks

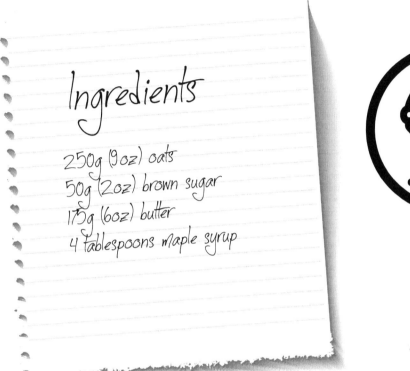

Ingredients

250g (9oz) oats
50g (2oz) brown sugar
175g (6oz) butter
4 tablespoons maple syrup

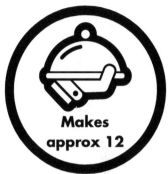

Makes approx 12

Method

Line a small shallow baking tin with greaseproof paper. Place the butter, sugar and syrup in a saucepan and stir until the sugar has dissolved then remove from the heat. Add the oats and mix well. Transfer the oats to the baking tin and smooth them down. Bake in the oven at 180C/360F for 25 minutes until golden. Allow to cool slightly and cut into squares. Wait until the flapjacks are cool before removing them from the tin.

Chocolate Milkshake

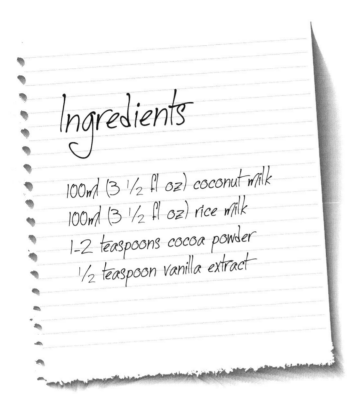

Ingredients

100ml (3 ½ fl oz) coconut milk
100ml (3 ½ fl oz) rice milk
1-2 teaspoons cocoa powder
½ teaspoon vanilla extract

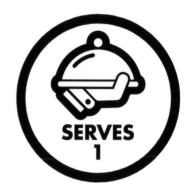

SERVES
1

Method

Place all the ingredients into a blender and process until smooth and frothy. Enjoy!
You can reduce the amount of coconut milk and replace it with extra rice milk or even
almond milk if you prefer. Alternatively, replace the cocoa powder with strawberries or
banana.

Orange & Raspberry Fruity Water

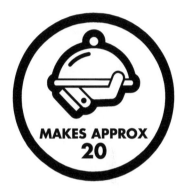

MAKES APPROX 20

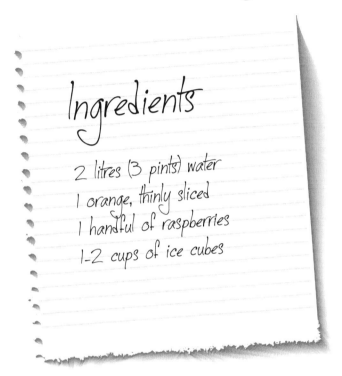

Ingredients

2 litres (3 pints) water
1 orange, thinly sliced
1 handful of raspberries
1-2 cups of ice cubes

Method

A great replacement for fizzy, sugary drinks is fruit infused water. Fill a glass jug with water, add a small amount of fruit together with some ice and refrigerate it for 2-3 hours. You will only need a small amount of fruit, even less for stronger ingredients such a fennel and herbs. Experiment with some of these tasty combinations:

Cucumber & Mint, Orange & Lime, Strawberry & Lime, Pineapple & Raspberry, Kiwi & Lemon, Lime & Cucumber, Orange & Thyme, Orange & Ginger, Lemon & Mint, Pineapple & Passion fruit.

Roast Mixed Nuts

SERVES 6

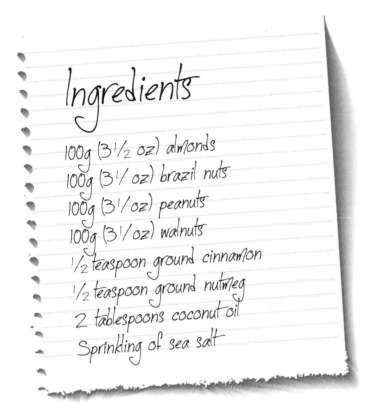

Ingredients

100g (3½ oz) almonds
100g (3½ oz) brazil nuts
100g (3½ oz) peanuts
100g (3½ oz) walnuts
½ teaspoon ground cinnamon
½ teaspoon ground nutmeg
2 tablespoons coconut oil
Sprinkling of sea salt

Method

Heat the coconut oil in a large frying pan. Add the nuts, cinnamon, nutmeg and salt.
Stir constantly for around 7-8 minutes. Store or serve as a party nibble or snack.

Courgette (Zucchini) Chips

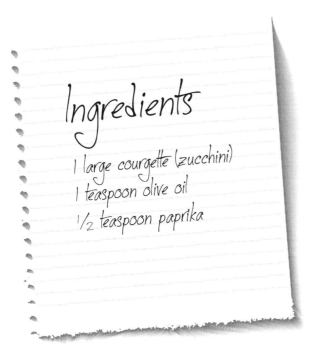

Ingredients

1 large courgette (zucchini)
1 teaspoon olive oil
1/2 teaspoon paprika

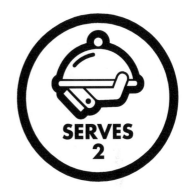

SERVES
2

Method

Slice the courgette (zucchini) into thin circles, around the thickness of a coin. Place them in a bowl, add a teaspoon of olive oil and paprika. Toss to lightly coat them. Line a baking sheet with foil, and lay out the slices onto the sheet. Preheat the oven to 220C/425F. Bake the chips for 30 minutes. Remove when crispy and golden. Serve and eat immediately.

Wheat-Free Chicken Stock (Broth)

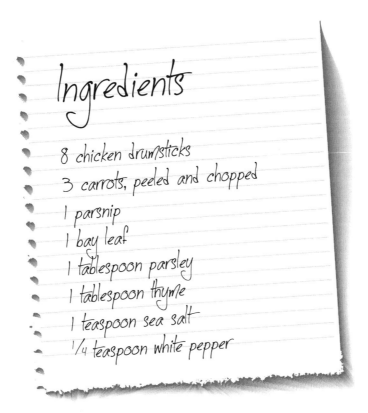

Ingredients

8 chicken drumsticks
3 carrots, peeled and chopped
1 parsnip
1 bay leaf
1 tablespoon parsley
1 tablespoon thyme
1 teaspoon sea salt
1/4 teaspoon white pepper

Method

Place all the ingredients into a large soup saucepan, cover with the water and bring to the boil. Reduce to a low heat. Skim off any foam from the top of the pot. Simmer for 90 minutes. Allow to cool then strain the stock (broth) through a sieve and place in containers ready to be frozen. Use a draining spoon and remove the chicken. It can be saved and made into a curry or kept as a leftover meal to be added to stir fries or omelettes.

For vegetable stock remove the chicken and substitute it for some courgette, spinach and pumpkin.

Tomato & Red Pepper Salsa

Ingredients

4 ripe tomatoes, deseeded and chopped
1 red pepper (bell pepper), finely chopped
4 spring onions (scallions), green part only, finely chopped
Handful of fresh coriander (cilantro) leaves, chopped
Juice of 1 lime

Method

Place the red pepper (bell pepper) under a hot grill (broiler) and cook until the skin blisters. Place the pepper in a bowl and cover with plastic wrap for 2 minutes to help bring the skin off and then peel it. Discard the skin and chop the flesh. Combine the pepper in a bowl with the chopped tomatoes, coriander (cilantro) and green part of the spring onions. Add the juice of the lime and season with salt and pepper

Tomato & Herb Sauce

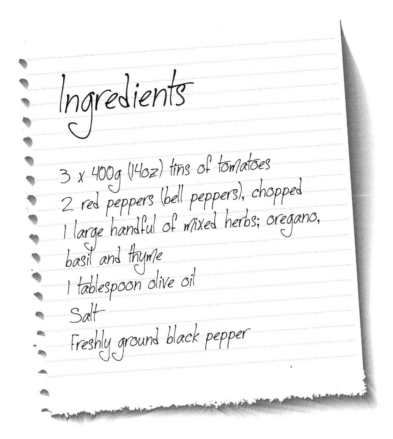

Ingredients

3 x 400g (14oz) tins of tomatoes
2 red peppers (bell peppers), chopped
1 large handful of mixed herbs; oregano,
basil and thyme
1 tablespoon olive oil
Salt
Freshly ground black pepper

Method

Heat the olive oil in a pan. Add the red pepper (bell pepper) and cook until soft. Pour in the tomatoes and cook for 15 minutes. Add the mixed herbs and season with salt and pepper. This makes a large batch which can be frozen and used for sauces and pizza toppings.

Printed in Great Britain
by Amazon